Alzheimer's

Dementia & Memory Loss

Help ME cope & survive!

STRAIGHT TALK FOR FAMILIES AND CAREGIVERS

MONICA VEST WHEELER

ISBN 978-0-9759875-4-4

A portion of the proceeds from the sale of this book will be donated to the Alzheimer's Association, Central Illinois Chapter.

**Help is available 24 hours a day, 7 days a week.
24-hour Hotline: 1-800-272-3900**

Alzheimer's Association, Central Illinois Chapter

Peoria office	Quincy area office	Rock River office
606 W. Glen Ave.	639 York St. Rm. 200	93 S. Hennepin Ave.
Peoria, IL 61614	Quincy, IL 62301	Dixon, IL 61021
Phone: 309-681-1100	Phone: 217-228-1111	Phone: 815-285-1100
Fax: 309-681-1101	Fax: 217-592-3690	Fax: 815-285-1116

Contact BF Press to find out how you can sell this book as a fundraiser for your organization or to buy in bulk.

BF Press
P.O. Box 3065
Peoria, IL 61612-3065
Toll-free 877-267-4640 (877-COPING-0)
www.bfpress.com

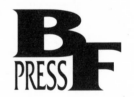

Contact us online and order additional books at:
www.alzhelpbook.com or www.bfpress.com

The
Help ME Cope & Survive!
series concept was created by
Joy Erlichman Miller, Ph.D., and Monica Vest Wheeler
with Diane Cullinan Oberhelman in
Cancer: Here's How YOU Can Help ME Cope & Survive
www.cancerhelpbook.com

What's inside

5
Author's note

8
Terms to remember

9
How to use this book

11
When Alzheimer's, dementia
or memory loss invades

12 In her own words
13 Alzheimer's 101
16 Warning signs
21 "Losing my best friend"
23 "The brain has a disease"
24 Hard questions
25 Why should I help?
29 An "ordinary" conversation
30 Just talking …
34 Everyday adjustments
35 In her own words
38 "Step on toes if you have to"
41 "You never never argue"
42 Research many sources
48 "No one believed me"
50 "She'd mask it and we'd
   say never mind"
58 Just talking …

62 Talking to the doctor
63 "What about …"
64 Dealing with doctors
74 From reaction to action

75
The necessities &
wisdom of planning

79 Financial and legal health
84 Stop the flow of money
88 Proactive or procrastinate?
90 What is HIPAA all about?
92 Paper piles
94 "We need to prepare for our
   own longevity"
98 One family's on-the-job lessons

99
Coping: It's full of trials
& errors & successes

100 Just talking …
103 Acceptance isn't easy
108 "I get frustrated and he gets
    mad at me"
110 Adapting to new realities
112 For the record
116 In her own words
117 Everyday realities
118 "Take your special moments,
    cherish them to the fullest"

*This book is being made available
to families through the generosity of
Valerie Dickson
and the Alzheimer's Association,
Central Illinois Chapter*

4

126 Just talking …
132 "We're affected by all this but you aren't — why?"
136 Just talking …
138 Taking away the car keys
140 Educating the public

141
Making adjustments

142 In his own words
143 "See what all he used to be able to do?"
150 "I don't see Dad as a guy with Alzheimer's"
160 Just talking …

163
Discovering & rediscovering the beauty of everyday life

164 No more excuses!
166 Digging not-so-deep
167 Making those memories
168 History 101
169 Stirring up memories
170 Rediscover their history
174 Creativity and patience

174
Asking for & accepting assistance

178 Just talking …
182 Caregivers must pay attention to their own needs
190 There are no stereotypes
199 Dealing with relatives
200 Build your team without screaming
214 Support groups
216 Letter to family & friends

217
The tough side of transitions

222 A matter of survival
225 One way to stop a thief
228 "She thought I was stealing things"
231 A letter to my loved one
232 Role changes require patience
237 "I am still dating my wife"
242 "Keep them engaged and going for as long as possible"
245 Caregiving without guilt
256 Dig for the humor
260 "I'm not sure if I would change anything"

263
Saying good-bye

264 Letting go
276 "I couldn't figure it out"

285
Looking back

297 Just talking …

299
A not-so-final note

303
Credits & resources

Please note: This book does not make nor attempt to make any diagnosis or suggest any specific treatment regarding any personal physical or emotional issues. Nor does it make or attempt to make any specific recommendations regarding financial or legal matters. Contact a certified and competent professional to address any concerns.

Alzheimer's has a face: our loved one

Read it, write in it, embrace it, refer to it any time of the day or night, tear pages out, pass it along, throw it on the floor in anger and frustration.

Better to hit the book than yourself or someone you love.

Alzheimer's, dementia and memory loss have become all-too-common words in our modern vocabulary. How long these disorders have been part of the human experience is hard to say because overall we're healthier and living longer than ever before.

The Alzheimer's Association estimates that more than 5 *million* Americans have Alzheimer's disease, twice as many as were diagnosed in 1980. Since then, this disease, named for the groundbreaking work of Dr. Alois Alzheimer, has acquired a face ... prominent public figures like President Ronald Reagan, actress Rita Hayworth, artist Norman Rockwell, boxer Sugar Ray Robinson, author E.B. White.

And people closer to our hearts ... our spouses, parents, grandparents, siblings and friends.

Alzheimer's, a form of dementia, and memory loss are *not* normal progressions of the aging process. Most individuals enter their senior years vital and connected to the world around them. However, these disorders rob millions of the basic ability to communicate and interact with those they love. It saddens and sickens family and friends who witness the hideous and hidden breakdown of the brain cells that define us as human beings ... the substance that has made us unique and special somebodies to others.

While these conditions are not good news, they are something you can cope with and survive in caring for a loved one.

This book isn't a dissertation about dementia and memory loss, but it does offer an insight into their everyday realities, and that's where Alzheimer's does it real damage. It's a

"Mentioning Alzheimer's is a conversation stopper." John, 59, mother, Alzheimer's

guidebook for loved ones and friends in coping with and surviving the challenges, heartaches and rewards these conditions bring. You won't find medical advice, yet I will guarantee you'll discover an abundance of human experiences, advice and life lessons that will reassure you that, while your circumstances and relationships are genuinely unique, you certainly are not alone. It's not easy reading at times, but it reinforces the healthy need to communicate with our loved ones and friends.

6

I learned so much from and am forever grateful to those dozens of caregivers who took the time to complete a comprehensive survey for this volume on how they've been affected emotionally and physically by the diagnosis of a loved one with dementia or memory loss. Their words and insights are an incredible description of their world and how they're confronting these irreversible and debilitating diseases. Their lessons must be shared with those coping with similar circumstances.

Thanks to the devoted and enthusiastic staff at the Alzheimer's Association, Central Illinois Chapter, I was given an extraordinary in-depth look into the who-what-when-where of memory loss and dementia and a fraction of the millions of lives affected by these brutal diseases.

Alzheimer's has a human face … our loved one.

For nearly a year and a half, I had a unique opportunity to attend educational and support group meetings for newly diagnosed clients and their immediate caregivers as they began their journey. They could only imagine what the future would bring.

Nothing or no one could have prepared me for what *I* would experience.

I listened, I learned, I laughed, I wept without shame. The families I have come to know and love accepted me with open minds and arms. They welcomed me into their homes and hearts. They shared and confided their joys and sorrows,

"I thought she was being irresponsible out of orneriness. She had a small tumor I thought was responsible for her behavior. It turned out to be Alzheimer's." Kevin, 45, mother, Alzheimer's

"It would be harder on us than it ever would be on him." Andrew, 25, father, frontal lobe dementia, diagnosed at age 51

hopes and fears, gifts and losses. They didn't ask me to leave during a tough moment or an intense conversation.

Nothing could be more gratifying and humbling than their trust from the start, all of which lifted *me*, despite the fact that *they're* the ones living this nightmare every day.

Tissues are cheap. Human connections are priceless.

Those Alzheimer's Association sessions were so basic and beneficial, and that's why excerpts from those moments are featured throughout this book under the heading of "Just talking." These individuals simply communicated with each other in search of a common knowledge and understanding, which is all they want ... except for an immediate cure for dementia and memory loss before they lose one more moment of their loved ones' lives.

During my conversations with those diagnosed with dementia or memory loss in the early-mid stages, I listened to what they tried to express through an increasing veil of frustration and loss that time cruelly manipulates with every passing hour. You'll find these exchanges on pages appropriately titled, "In her/his own words."

I quickly learned that no matter what individuals with dementia and memory loss try to articulate at whatever stage, and even if what we hear is garbled and confused, they still deserve the dignity of being heard. We must take the time to sit beside them, hold their hand and look into their eyes and reassure them that we have not forgotten them ... though their minds and bodies may have forgotten us.

However, we know their spirits will never forget that immeasurable gesture of love. Neither will ours.

Monica Vest Wheeler

Terms to remember

Here are definitions of words, provided by the Alzheimer's Association, that you'll find referenced frequently in this book.

▸ **Alzheimer's disease** — *A disease of the brain that causes problems with memory, thinking and behavior. It is not a normal part of aging.*

▸ **Dementia** — *General term for the loss of memory and other intellectual abilities serious enough to interfere with daily life. Alzheimer's is the most common form of dementia.*

▸ **Memory loss** — *While clearly remembering things that happened long ago, someone with memory loss may quickly forget recent events, which may include trouble keeping track of time, people and places, forgetting appointments or people's names, forgetting where they put things.*

▸ **Mild cognitive impairment** — *Although a person may have noticeable difficulty with memory or other thinking skills, a doctor may determine the person does not meet criteria for being diagnosed with Alzheimer's or another form of dementia. It does not always mean the person will develop Alzheimer's.*

▸ **Early-onset** — *A type of Alzheimer's disease that affects people who are under age 65. Many are in their 40s and 50s. Up to 10 percent of people with Alzheimer's have this kind.*

▸ **Early-stage** — *The early part of Alzheimer's when problems with memory and concentration may begin to appear in a doctor's interview or medical tests.*

▸ **Dementia with Lewy Body** — *Often starts with wide variations in attention and alertness. Individuals affected by this illness often experience visual hallucinations as well as muscle rigidity and tremors similar to those associated with Parkinson's disease.*

▸ **Frontotemporal dementia or Pick's disease** — *Rare disorder that may sometimes be hard to distinguish from Alzheimer's. Personality changes and disorientation often occur before memory loss.*

▸ **MedicAlert+Alzheimer's Association Safe Return** — *A program that issues identification products that include a toll-free 24-hour emergency response number to reunite a family and a person with dementia who wanders or becomes lost.*

- **Sundowning** — *When persons with Alzheimer's experience periods of increased confusion, anxiety, agitation and disorientation beginning at dusk and continuing throughout the night.*

- **Vascular dementia** — *Impairment caused by reduced blood flow to parts of the brain.*

- **HIPAA** — *Health Insurance Portability and Accountability Act.*

- **Power of attorney (POA)** — *Allows the person with dementia to name an individual to make financial decisions when he or she is no longer able (considered legally incompetent).*

- **Durable power of attorney** — *The power of attorney document is valid even after the person with dementia can no longer make decisions for himself or herself.*

- **Power of attorney for health care** — *Allows a person to name an individual to act on his or her behalf to make health care decisions when he or she is no longer able.*

- **CT** — *Computed tomography*

- **MRI** — *Magnetic resonance imaging*

- **PET** — *Positron emission tomography*

- **Transient ischemic attack (TIA)** — *A temporary loss of brain function and a warning sign for a possible future stroke.*

How to use this book

This volume is composed of numerous elements to provide you with a variety of useful insights and tools in coping with the everyday challenges of Alzheimer's, dementia and memory loss.

You'll find short statements from caregivers who responded to a detailed survey in dealing with all stages. Through short stories and the special "In his/her own words" and "Just talking," you'll be introduced to individuals who share their experiences in more detail. You'll also discover how families coped with specific challenges via snippets of advice or venting of frustrations.

Most topics are only one to three pages in length to make it easier for you to pick up and put down as *your* time and energy permits. You'll also find spaces to jot your thoughts or reminders that will help you get through difficult situations.

Use the ideas or suggestions presented here as springboards for ways to cope with and survive *your* unique circumstances.

An ordinary day until...

You're going through the motions of everyday life: You work, play, sleep, eat, love, celebrate, get frustrated, interact with people, spend time alone, fulfill financial responsibilities, tackle challenges, cherish old memories and create new ones.

Much of life is automatic, like breathing, knowing when to eat, sleep and follow a personal hygiene regimen. Your body knows how to respond to rituals like household chores, driving, reading and common courtesies and manners on its own without thinking or prompting.

However, one day, we notice something different about a loved one, something that has been nagging at us ... *Yes, they've been doing that for a while ... No, they've never behaved that way before.* When asked, many caregivers explained that they had noticed changes but had not tried nor wanted to discover the source of the problem.

Why? Because human beings do not invite bad news even when we know something is wrong. We hope that if we ignore it, it will go away.

At moments like this, we can't decide which cliché is more appropriate ... *The truth will set you free* ... or ... *The truth hurts.*

"I started to notice a difference in her. She didn't seem to want to be around others. She was quieter than usual. It could have been earlier when I look back. People change, and I did not pay enough attention." Robert, 79, wife, Alzheimer's, died 6 years after diagnosed

When Alzheimer's, dementia or memory loss invades YOUR world

"I found a note he'd written much later, but he said in very misspelled, grammatically incorrect words that he had been diagnosed with Alzheimer's, and it had affected both his quality and enjoyment of life."
Ann, 49, mother, vascular dementia; father, Alzheimer's

In her own words

Denise noticed changes in her 80-something mother when her father died several years ago, but it wasn't until later that things became obvious.

The daughter wonders aloud if her father had covered up for her mother, Wilma, who tells this visitor, "Nah." The father had a stroke during an operation.

"He didn't know me. He'd run away," Wilma recalls, shaking her head. "I'd have to go look for him. I slept on a chair by the front door so he couldn't go out. I wasn't getting any rest. It wasn't good for me either. You get stressed out about things, and you 'lose it,' you really do. I do all right here."

Denise smiles. "You can talk to her on the phone. You can talk to her here, and she's just fine. But she was fooling us a lot" as the episodes of forgetfulness increased in frequency.

Wilma jumps back into the conversation. "I don't forget to get up in the morning. I don't forget to eat."

When asked why she attends educational and support group meetings at the local chapter of the Alzheimer's Association, Wilma turns to her youngest daughter and asks her why she's going. Before Denise answers, her mother speaks again.

"I remember to get up. I remember to go to bed. I know, I forget things." She doesn't consider it frustrating though names escape her at times. "I forgot what I forget." She smiles.

"I drove up until I got rid of my car. Not that I didn't want to drive. I think everybody wanted me to quit." She chuckles. "They felt safer out there if I didn't drive. I just quit. I didn't care to be around these people who are driving today. I figured I was safer walking." She passed a driving test a year earlier. Smiling, she reminds her daughter that "*they* weren't afraid." However, "it's so nice to hitch a ride with your daughter.

"Nobody from church offered to come by and pick me up. So, I don't go." Why not? "I don't like to ask people to do anything or go out of their way for me. But I'd go out of my way for anybody else."

Alzheimer's 101: Introducing families to basics of the disease

This session could have been called "Alzheimer's 101," but Alisha, the young professional leading the discussion, opts for a more formal title, "Facing New Challenges: An Understanding of Alzheimer's Disease." The 16 individuals in attendance don't care what name seasons it because they're too hungry for answers about this confusing disease that has intruded their lives.

This was a new workshop offered by the Alzheimer's Association, Central Illinois Chapter in response to the growing number of calls seeking basic information. The number in attendance this early fall evening exceeds the staff's expectations.

As patient and family services coordinator, Alisha reassures these sons, daughters, wives, husbands and siblings that just because everyone forgets things occasionally, it doesn't mean everyone has dementia or memory loss. Most nod at her example of how forgetting where we parked our car is okay, but forgetting what a car is used for is not.

Dementia and memory loss are not senility or the old-fashioned "hardening of the arteries" term. Alzheimer's is the most prevalent among the more than 70 types of irreversible dementia. Observers will often notice warning signs long before the individual will. (*A list of the 10 most prevalent signs of Alzheimer's is on page 16*).

Age remains the greatest risk factor. An estimated one in 10 at age 65 will have some form of dementia or memory loss. That figure jumps to one in two at age 85. More women have Alzheimer's, and family history is also a risk. Alisha says that's why there is a huge concern over how this disease will affect society as the baby boomers age.

"Every 72 seconds, someone develops Alzheimer's. By 2050, an estimated *16 million* will have it," she explains.

While these conditions were much harder to officially diagnose even a decade ago, medical advances in CT and PET scans now enable a clearer look at the brain, which often shrinks and creates caverns as the disease progresses. A protein found in the brains of these individuals with Alzheimer's literally gums up the brain cells with plaque, which slows and disrupts the connections necessary for normal brain function.

A woman raises her hand and points to the projector screen.

"Why does it say fatal?"

Alisha composes her answer.

"Alzheimer's lasts three to 20 years. Families call and ask how much time they've got. A very healthy person can live with it for a very long time. In later stages, which is far down the road, we aren't able to walk anymore. We probably could physically do it, but our brain doesn't remember how to." With Alzheimer's, the last skills lost are generally those learned earliest in life, if the patient has not succumbed to pneumonia or another malady first.

Glancing around the silent room, she continues.

"That's a real downer. This is not an up disease. We're not excited about it, but what I'm excited about is that if we catch it earlier, we can have a longer quality of life. That's why it's important to get to the doctor."

While current medications do not slow the degenerative process, Alisha explains, they can extend the period of more cognitive awareness and buy precious time during which the individuals can be involved more in their future plans. This also allows the family to prepare emotionally and financially.

She stresses that legal and financial issues cannot be ignored with this type of diagnosis. She recommends that everyone have a living will and other affairs in order to make it easier on the family, no matter whether it's Alzheimer's or any other circumstance.

In addition, many individuals, if diagnosed early enough, can continue to take care of themselves for a long time. However, family and friends need to be attuned to matters such as safety, driving and finances, and make sure the person is not exploited or in danger. Unfortunately, she adds, there are no clear markers of being incapacitated because everyone and every case is different.

"This is not a black and white disease," Alisha says.

Someone asks about driving.

Alisha explains that a diagnosis of Alzheimer's does not mean an automatic removal of driving privileges.

"Would you trust them with *your* child? That's the question."

Each person has to weigh the pros and cons of telling extended family or friends about a dementia or memory loss diagnosis.

She explains that it can help educate others and put everyone at ease with knowledge. However, some people are afraid of negative stereotypes and the risk of social isolation.

"You can't change the disease. You *can* change *your* attitude."

Loved ones should remember that research shows that 55 percent of communication is non-verbal body language, 38 percent is pitch and tone, and only 7 percent is verbal. This is especially crucial in interacting with individuals with dementia and memory loss.

Alisha explains that supportive listening is paying attention while someone speaks. Since our eyes tell much about us, look them in the eye. See where they're looking to help identify what they may be unable to verbalize. Be aware of what distractions may interrupt their efforts to communicate.

For example, the individuals eventually have trouble talking on the phone because their brains can no longer understand the abstract concept of voices carried over phone lines or an intercom.

It's not uncommon for people with Alzheimer's to be afraid of making mistakes, she says. Reverting to a fear they may have experienced as a child being called upon in class, it may prompt them to stop talking all together. Consider these quick tips:

- *Say the person's name to get their attention.*
- *Don't challenge or correct them. If they say the sky is red, then let it be red. However, you might want to question them if they want to wear shorts in the middle of winter.*
- *Maintain a sense of humor no matter what.*
- *Avoid arguing, giving orders or over-simplifying something unless it's a safety issue.*
- *If they have trouble deciding on something to do, give them something purposeful so they feel as if they're making a contribution.*
- *And most importantly, don't set them up for failure.*

As she concludes her presentation, she reminds them to "create meaningful moments."

10 warning signs of Alzheimer's

Courtesy of Alzheimer's Association www.alz.org

1 **Memory loss.** Forgetting recently learned information is one of the most common early signs of dementia. A person begins to forget more often and is unable to recall the information later.

What's normal? Forgetting names or appointments occasionally.

2 **Difficulty performing familiar tasks.** People with dementia often find it hard to plan or complete everyday tasks. Individuals may lose track of the steps involved in preparing a meal, placing a telephone call or playing a game.

What's normal? Occasionally forgetting why you came into a room or what you planned to say.

3 **Problems with language.** People with Alzheimer's disease often forget simple words or substitute unusual words, making their speech or writing hard to understand. They may be unable to find the toothbrush, for example, and instead ask for "that thing for my mouth."

What's normal? Sometimes having trouble finding the right word.

4 **Disorientation to time and place.** People with Alzheimer's disease can become lost in their own neighborhood, forget where they are, how they got there, and not know how to get back home.

What's normal? Forgetting the day of the week or where you were going.

5 **Poor or decreased judgment.** Individuals with Alzheimer's may dress inappropriately, wearing several layers on a warm day or little clothing in the cold. They may show poor judgment, like giving away large sums of money to telemarketers.

What's normal? Making a questionable or debatable decision from time to time.

6 **Problems with abstract thinking.** Someone with Alzheimer's disease may have unusual difficulty performing complex mental tasks, like forgetting what numbers are for and how they should be used.

What's normal? Finding it challenging to balance a checkbook.

7 **Misplacing things.** A person with Alzheimer's disease may put things in unusual places: an iron in the freezer or a wristwatch in the sugar bowl.

What's normal? Misplacing keys or a wallet temporarily.

8 **Changes in mood or behavior.** Someone with Alzheimer's disease may show rapid mood swings – from calm to tears to anger – for no apparent reason.

What's normal? Occasionally feeling sad or moody.

9 **Changes in personality.** The personalities of people with dementia can change dramatically. They may become extremely confused, suspicious, fearful or dependent on a family member.

What's normal? Personalities do change somewhat with age.

10 **Loss of initiative.** A person with Alzheimer's may become very passive, sitting in front of the TV for hours, sleeping more than usual or not wanting to do usual activities.

What's normal? Sometimes feeling weary of work or social obligations.

Caregivers say...

Part of this role we play as human beings is being immersed in relationships of all types with family and friends ... close and distant, emotionally and physically ... rewarding and challenging ... simply good and bad. No two human connections are the same. Nobody's perfect, but there are individuals in our lives who we feel are pretty close to earning that status, people who seem to be part of every breath we take.

Describe your relationship with this person before the diagnosis, i.e. close, casual, estranged, and in what way

- Close
- Lived in the same city
- Only child in this state
- Close but not part of each other's everyday life
- Dutiful daughter
- Loving and compatible couple for 50 years
- Relationship mixed
- Shared sons and disagreements
- Loved each other very much

- Very close-knit family
- Talk by phone weekly
- Major family get-togethers at parents' home
- Preparing for a happy retirement together
- Not close
- No intimacy
- He has a repressive personality
- Did everything together

- We were always close and would always help each other in whatever was needed. I miss her very much. *Jolene, 66, mother, dementia, died 5 years after diagnosed*

- Close and loving. My folks lived two hours away, but we saw them frequently (once or twice a month). After Mom had bypass surgery, we moved them to the town where we live. *Ann, 49, mother, vascular dementia, died; father, Alzheimer's, died*

- We were close. We did things together. She was part of my life. *Kim, 34, grandmother, died 5 years after diagnosed*

18

- I was always the one she felt safe to tell things. She shared with me before she was diagnosed that she was having trouble with her bills and did not understand how to take her meds. *Jenny, 56, mother, Alzheimer's*

- His head injury happened in 1971. We were married 20 years with small children. *Roseann, 72, husband, dementia, died 10 years after diagnosed*

19

- Close, honest with each other, loyal, great love for one another, loved our family, cared for others (like both of our parents), dined out and danced, lots of dancing, and faith in God. *Robert, 79, wife, Alzheimer's, died 6 years after diagnosed*

- We were never close. She was not truthful and would deny it. She never took care of anything. Poor parenting skills. *Elaine, 54, mother, Alzheimer's*

- My mother was fiercely independent in the 17 years after my father died. She seldom asked for help or needed it. She always came to family birthday celebrations and holiday gatherings, but otherwise she enjoyed her own circle of friends. *Judith, 61, mother, Alzheimer's*

- Fairly close. Mother was domineering. I had learned how to handle her and my own life. She was also totally deaf the last 10 years of her life, which made for special challenges and empathy. *Anne, 67, mother, dementia, died 4 years after diagnosed*

- My husband and I were self-employed together for 20-plus years. We really were best friends. *Vicky, 54, husband, early onset Alzheimer's, died 5 years after diagnosed*

- Very close. I was very fortunate to have such a wonderful father. I cherish the memories and time spent together. *Andrew, 25, father, frontal lobe dementia, diagnosed at age 51*

"My grandma and I were very close. I would help her with daily activities, and she would give me a shoulder to cry on when I was upset." *Shallen, 25, grandmother, Alzheimer's*

▶ I've always been close to my parents. When my father passed away, I naturally stepped in to care for my mom. *Sally, 57, mother, Alzheimer's, died 3 years after diagnosed*

▶ We were happily married for over 50 years and were inseparable. *Bill, 78, wife, Alzheimer's, died 4 years after diagnosed*

> "One never got close to Mother. She was a closed person. She never kissed me or told me she loved me." Nancy, 65, mother, Alzheimer's

▶ Married almost 40 years. He has always had trouble expressing himself. Quiet, kind, hard-working. *Sandy, 61, husband, Alzheimer's and vascular dementia*

▶ Extremely close. She is my best friend, the greatest mom in the world. *Kevin, 45, mother, Alzheimer's*

▶ Close. We do most everything together, traveled. Our children and their families get together with friends and families. *Norma, 81, husband, Alzheimer's*

▶ My mom was close to my children, and she was close to me, not only as Mom, but as my best friend. We did everything together. *MM, 46, mother, Alzheimer's, died 5 years after diagnosed*

> "Always close, still close. I honor and respect him and want to maintain his dignity." Mary Ann, 62, father, Alzheimer's

▶ Very close, like a mother. *J, grandmother, Alzheimer's*

Losing "my best friend"

Denise's eyes follow her mother, Wilma, as she walks back to the kitchen to watch a favorite TV show, "Jeopardy." Alzheimer's is stealing the mind and body of the woman she's always admired and adored.

"She was my best friend. I could tell my mom anything, and I still can, but there's no reply. It's not there anymore." When Mom does answer, it's all about *her* now as Wilma's world has shrunk. "So, I can tell her anything, pour my heart out to her, and her reply is, 'I wonder what I'm going to do today.' That has hurt a lot." It's probably been a year and half since they've had a meaningful two-way conversation.

The events of recent months had added to the emotional emptiness as the daughter, youngest of four adult children, had battled cancer. How has her mom responded to the diagnosis?

"She says, 'It doesn't run in our family. I never had it.' That's all she says every time. It's hard. I'm the one taking it the hardest. She was always there for me. She watched my kids when I worked. She and Dad went to all my kids' games ...

"It broke my heart at first, and I cried all the time. My siblings got sick of me calling all the time crying. It's made me stronger, and I think that's how I've gotten through the cancer. If I had had cancer four or five years ago, I don't think I would have been as strong as I am now.

"A few years ago, Mom gave me power-of-attorney because she said I was the only one she could trust to not put her in a home before her time." She smiles. "And she's right, as long as I think she can handle it here." Someone helps with cleaning, shoveling and other chores. Denise worries about how she will adjust to assisted living in the future and is afraid her health will fail.

"A (nursing) home is definitely the last thing I want to do. She still plays cards and is happy. Why take that away from her ... or me? I'll be selfish as long as she can play cards, laugh and have a good time. I can see her being bitter if that's taken away. She's still stubborn and always has been.

"I call her three-four times a day to make sure she's eating and taking her medicine. She only cooks in the microwave now. She hates frozen dinners, but when it comes to dinner time, she opens the freezer and says, 'I have these lovely dinners.' The microwave and the TV, those are the last two things she can barely work around here."

22

She's carefully observed the changes in her mother and made adjustments along the way, including building in more time in getting Wilma ready to leave the house. She's not fond of baths anymore and only allows Denise or her hairdresser to wash her hair.

"She looks forward to Chicago Cubs games. I told her they were on the radio. She couldn't remember what a radio was the other day. That just devastated me. I had to explain what it was, and she figured out, 'Oh, I do have two or three of them.' "

Wilma often tells the same story and never deviates.

"I don't know if it's really true anymore, and the memories used to be more in-depth than now. That scares me, too. I mention things she might remember, but they're gone."

She used to work all the newspaper puzzles, but that hobby ceased about a year ago. She used to love soap operas but can't follow them anymore. She's been having trouble with names, including some of the grandchildren and great-grandchildren. Denise once found in a drawer about 30 checks that had not been mailed. She can't figure out the mail anymore.

"The way the memory works … it's just such a mystery."

Wilma spends most of her time in the kitchen.

"I think she feels safe there. Her world is getting smaller. She doesn't even go upstairs." The daughter found the middle leaf of the table gone one day to make the dining room table smaller.

"Nobody gives you a list or a test of what you need to look into."

Returning to the dining room, Wilma hugs her baby.

"I thought I was through having children, then along came Denise. She was a blessing. She's a blessing. Isn't she sweet? Does she look anything like me? Only she's prettier. She's younger, that's why. When I was young, I was pretty. Then of course, you get old and lose it." She laughs all the way back to the kitchen.

"I love her," Denise says. "I'm going to do everything I can for her. She brought me into this world, and she's not going out of this world anytime before I let her. It's taught me more patience and strength. I think I'm strong enough to get through anything … except for totally losing her."

"The brain has a disease"

With a background in the mental health field, Bonnie has assisted families coping with dementia and memory loss at the Alzheimer's Association for a decade. She's discovered that many don't understand that dementia is a physical illness. It's often thrown in the "wrong basket." Individuals are usually told to concentrate harder. " 'It'll be better.' It won't. The brain has a disease."

Unfortunately, this education specialist finds that any disorder related to the brain still carries a stigma. Dementia patients on television or in the movies are often portrayed as manic, which is the rarity. The 1 percent gets all the attention.

"What's interesting is that the people with dementia, many don't realize anything is wrong with them. The memory loss and problems have been slow and gradual. She has her memories, so she thinks she's doing all these things we know she's not doing. It's like the teenage years. Some glide through, some go kicking and screaming. Other people have more of an awareness that there is something wrong."

Bonnie remembers asking one family member, "What was the reaction to the diagnosis?" It was relief, because now they knew something was actually wrong. It's a physical, medical disease, something people cannot control.

With individuals who have more awareness, there is more fear, sadness and grief. "He may see his daughter walking down the aisle, but he may not realize it," she explains.

"The loss of the ability to think is far more frightening than the loss of the ability to use their bodies. There is a difference in the quality of life, that if I can at least understand it or I can talk … If I can't do those, it's scary."

How has she been affected by her work?

"I try to be more patient, definitely grateful. I feel so blessed to have this job. I really do believe that people touch us far more than we touch them."

She says there is this amazing connection, and it's interesting in this type of work that they don't ever truly know how they have reached out to someone, even if it's only one encounter. Sometimes the families only need one little piece of the map to get to the next place they need to go.

Hard questions...

"I was completely oblivious"

Her husband's odd behavior started a few years before he was diagnosed with early-onset Alzheimer's at age 59. Ignorant then of Alzheimer's and related disorders, Peg now admits, "I don't know why I didn't take him earlier." He had always been involved in insurance, real estate and appraisals. She first noticed he was having trouble doing his job, so she started helping him that last year he was able to work. She had always worked with him, "but I guess I was completely oblivious. Now when I look back, it was ridiculous, but I was."

He finally realized he was forgetting things and where he was going. He didn't forget people and faces, but always had trouble with names, so that forgetfulness didn't signal any problems. When he was finally diagnosed, it was easier when he started referring everything to Peg.

"Do you think I have Alzheimer's?"

Sue says: "My mother was driving by herself here, and she didn't come and didn't come. The phone rang. She had gotten lost. She was actually only two blocks away from my house. I got her there and then on to church. She leaned over and asked, 'Do you think I have Alzheimer's?' I said, 'Well …' So I started asking questions and found out from my dad that there were things happening; she was forgetting things. She would call me frequently with the same question.

"My father was killed in an accident. He was just telling me that he was getting concerned, finding bills thrown away. He must have been covering an awful lot. I had her evaluated, and they said it was early dementia, but there was no treatment. That was before some of the drugs they have now. So we kept an eye on her, and she functioned fairly well. I started going over every weekend, and then I realized it was so much worse than any of us had known."

Why should *I* help?

Not all relationships are loving, friendly and fulfilling. Sometimes they're uncomfortably strained, riddled with animosity or virtually non-existent for whatever reason. Other relationships are considered family on paper only or are a distant relative you had no time, interest or motivation in getting to know better.

However, what if *you* were called upon to help care for a family member with whom you had not been close, someone who has been diagnosed with dementia or memory loss? Or maybe an aunt, uncle or grandparent you hardly know? Or a parent who never said, "I love you"? Or a spouse you once loved but with whom now you share only a house?

How do we bridge or patch relationships to bear or survive a crisis? How do we put earlier conflicts in the past? How do we look for the best or at least something positive in someone? How do we get to know someone from scratch, someone for whose care we may be ultimately responsible?

Fear and love are often described as two of the greatest motivators in life. The former may become the more prevalent or obvious emotion when it comes to confronting the challenge of memory loss or an Alzheimer's diagnosis. Fear of loneliness and/or death can crack some of the toughest exteriors and interiors.

You never know who will ask for your assistance one day. You never know who *you* may need to call upon in a crisis. It's one of those "never-say-never" scenarios.

Ask yourself why you were "selected" to step in and care for an ailing relative. Are you the only one remaining in an older generation of a smaller extended family? Are you the only relative residing in the same community as the individual diagnosed? Are you the only adult child who's willing to help Mom or Dad? Are you the only one who didn't, who couldn't, say "no"? Does everyone assume you'll do everything because you're still married?

Ask yourself why you said "yes." Is it out of a sense of obligation? Guilt? A long-ago promise? Is it just the "right thing" to do because "we take care of our own"?

Even if you are not called upon to be the primary caregiver for a relative, you may have an opportunity to help initiate or mend a variety of relationships.

It's up to *you* whether it's a burden or opportunity.

Caregivers say...

Sometimes we're puzzled by someone's behavior, actions or comments that seem out of character. Not wanting to over-react, we often attribute it to a "bad day." We all have personality quirks and down days, but if these persist and the person's denial is too adamant, we can't help but question the source of these changes. Sometimes it's useful to document these events, so that *we* don't forget and to provide detailed information to medical personnel if necessary.

What symptoms or behavior did you notice about this person before they were diagnosed?

- Repeated himself
- Lost interest in grooming
- Couldn't find car in parking lot
- Called relatives several times a day
- Unable to pay bills
- Paid bills twice
- Wouldn't clean house
- Wouldn't wash clothes
- Poor health care
- Hair not combed
- Difficulty in completing small tasks
- Forgetfulness
- Confused
- Shuffled feet
- Fell often
- Got lost on familiar roads
- Acted differently

- Couldn't figure out numbers or time
- Awkward on telephone
- Angry at her best friends
- Uncertain of things
- Minor auto mishaps
- Doing things out of character
- Personality changes
- More demanding
- Took more risks
- Hid household bills
- Acted out
- Age regression
- Not eating properly
- Lost interest in things
- Failing memory
- Lack of motivation
- Disorganization
- Depression

▸ Confusion and halluci-
nations, seeing people
and things that were-
n't there. *Shallen, 25,
grandmother, Alzheimer's*

> "Became like an 'airhead,' not remembering." David, 69, wife, Alzheimer's

▸ My father "knew"
before his diagnosis
that he had trouble
remembering. *Ann, 49, mother, vascular
dementia, died; father, Alzheimer's, died*

▸ Some forgetfulness, repeating conversations. She would
have episodes of like going into a "stupor." *Jolene, 66, mother,
dementia, died 5 years after diagnosed*

▸ She was unable to fill out a check or write the date after 2000.
I just did not understand that. *Jenny, 56, mother, Alzheimer's*

▸ He couldn't remember where we kept things and couldn't
"catch on" to new information. *Leora, 72, husband, Alzheimer's*

▸ Both my mother and sister experienced loss of memory, how
to dress as to what color went with another. Giggled when
caught doing the wrong thing. Didn't remember important
dates or meetings. *Norma, 81, mother, Alzheimer's, died 11 years
after diagnosed; sister, Alzheimer's, died 6 years after diagnosed*

▸ Taking so long to complete a sentence. Slow thought process.
Nettie, 51, father, Alzheimer's

▸ Bladder incontinence, inappropriate dress. *Phil, 69, mother,
dementia*

▸ Quick temper, obsession with psychic phenomenon. *Roseann,
72, husband, dementia, died 10 years after diagnosed*

▸ Short memory, taking a light fixture and lamp apart to
change a light bulb. *Maxine,
77, husband, Alzheimer's*

> She bought thousands of things from TV shopping channels." Kevin, 45, mother, Alzheimer's

▸ Lack of reasoning and
common sense, recall of
certain family traditions
gone, forgetful. *June, 66,
husband, early onset Alz-
heimer's*

- We suggested she not drive. She was getting lost. She had greatly impaired judgment in financial matters and responded to every charitable mailing. *Judith, 61, mother, Alzheimer's*

- Utilities were disconnected and insurance cancelled for lack of payment. *Elaine, 54, mother, Alzheimer's*

- Severe depression, lack of interest in things important to her. *Nancy, 65, mother, Alzheimer's*

- Forgetfulness and self-limiting activities, such as travel, which she used to love. *Elizabeth, 47, mother, Alzheimer's*

- Lack of emotion, especially on September 11, 2001. No real reaction, disinterest and apathy. *Andrew, 25, father, frontal lobe dementia, diagnosed at age 51*

- A gradual loss of memory and function. *Bill, 78, wife, Alzheimer's, died 4 years after diagnosed*

- Holes in memory and getting angry at me. *Sandy, 61, husband, Alzheimer's and vascular dementia*

- Confusion, memory problems, sequence problems, not caring for herself. *Chris, 51, mother, Alzheimer's*

- Forgetful, unusual and unhealthy co-dependent relationship between my mom and grandmother after my father's death. *Jody, 47, mother, early onset Alzheimer's*

- Loss of memory. He told me back in 1996 he was "losing it." Mistakes on accounts, threw away important documents, files a mess. *Catherine, 85, husband, Alzheimer's and Lewy Body*

- Forgetting to switch off lights, where he put things (billfold and keys), repeating himself. *Norma, 81, husband, Alzheimer's*

- He actually became concerned himself when he couldn't remember things. *Helen, 72, husband, Alzheimer's*

"On my father's deathbed, he told me my mother was forgetful. I observed her and realized she could not be left alone." *Sally, 57, mother, Alzheimer's, died 3 years after diagnosed*

An "ordinary" conversation

Overheard ... an "ordinary" conversation between a husband with Alzheimer's and his wife ...

Wife: "Why are you so physically fit? Where do you drag me every single day, where I don't want to go?"

Husband: "What do we do? In the morning. Where are we?" He laughs.

Wife: "Where are we at 5 o'clock? Where did we go?"

Husband: "Yes, we did. We went someplace. Oh yeah. We went to the ..." While shaking his finger trying to remember, he grins.

Wife: "The gym."

Husband: "Yes, we go to the gym almost every day."

Wife: "We do *every* day. Not almost. I hate it with a passion though I know it's good for me." She vigorously shakes her head. "He's gone for years. You start slow and you work until it gets kind of boring. What's the first thing you do? Where do you go?"

Husband: "I go take off my shoes." He laughs again.

Wife: "Not your shoes. Your coat. What piece of equipment do you go to first?"

Husband: "Okay, piece of equipment, that's very, very easy. It is ... I don't know, what is it?"

Wife: "You walk. It's called a treadmill."

Husband: "Ah yes, treadmill. That is the first thing."

Wife: "Then where do we go?"

Husband: "After that, we go hide."

Wife: "You do that later. Where do you go after the treadmill? You sit down."

Husband: "I do?"

Wife: "You pedal. What's it called?"

Husband: "I don't know."

Wife: "You go on a bike."

Husband: "Stationary bike."

Wife: "Excellent! Then where do you go and hide?"

Husband: "I go and hide inside and work with you."

She says he goes on the toning table and sometimes falls asleep.

Wife: "Then you join me and what do we do in that room?"

Husband: "Nothing much."

Wife: "Geez, this is not a good day."

Husband: "I think we do well doing what we do. I'm satisfied with it."

Just talking...

(Caregiver and client responses and reactions are in italics.)

A question is posed to Alzheimer's Association facilitator Bonnie: *How do doctors know for sure that it's Alzheimer's?*

"It can be definitely diagnosed during an autopsy," she says.

When someone suggests that he's in no rush for an official diagnosis, the group laughs. This is an unconventional, yet interesting, icebreaker on the first night of this six-week educational and support group session for recently diagnosed clients and their immediate caregivers.

Ten pairs of memory loss or dementia clients and their primary caregivers relax in the large circle of chairs with facilitators Bonnie and Jenn. There's nothing extraordinary or ordinary about any of them, yet their life experiences and fears are as unique as their fingerprints …

Two couples have been married 49 years.

A mother pats the knees of her daughters sitting on either side of her. "These two look after me all the time. They think I'm 'it.' " *One daughter grins and says,* "Don't get her started." *Everyone laughs.*

One client's favorite hobby is riding his beloved horses.

Only in his early 50s, a dad lives by himself though knows that someday he won't be able to stay alone. His son and daughter reside in Chicago. "They're good kids," *he says. His sister reminds him,* "You're a good dad."

A husband with memory loss is reading mysteries and finds it stimulating, though it's hard to follow many characters.

One caregiver says her husband endured every test possible in search of answers. His body is in good condition; his mind isn't so good some days.

"I dragged him off the golf course to attend today," *says one wife. Her husband nods without a word.*

"In 49 years, this is the first thing he's agreed to do with me," *says another. Her spouse immediately answers,* "It was either this or divorce." *Everyone chuckles.*

A client says, "This is my wife, and she takes care of me. I get confused, but she straightens me out."

A daughter is here with her mother, though both parents have Alzheimer's. The mother acknowledges, "I belong here."

"I miss bowling," says one woman. "I'd go if somebody took me."

A man says that everything he needs is at home. "Everything there is valuable to me. It's the best place to be. I'm not going to go off and get things. I can't afford to go wandering."

Another acknowledges, "I get lost because of unfamiliar surroundings. All the mechanics work fine."

A client has been thinking about taking the bus more often, which is part of his new reality ...

Bonnie explains that dementia and memory loss are like a light bulb going on and off. Those rapid changes can be frustrating. One minute you're okay, but the next, it's like somebody pulled the plug. They're dealing with "little pieces of lost. It's hard for all of us when things change."

It's like a breeze when everyone nods.

It's hard to accept and explain such a diagnosis.

"People are private. We want to choose to whom we give information." She says that if she and someone from the group are out in public and see each other, she'll wait until they greet her first. The only exception to confidentiality is if individuals are in danger of harming themselves or others.

Is it okay to leave the client alone at home for short periods of time?

"It's a judgment call," says Bonnie. "There are no concrete rules. It all depends on the day and situation. Watch for signs of danger. You have to find a balance between quality of life and safety for everyone involved."

She advises them to look for signs just like they did when they left their children alone when they were old enough. All decisions must be based on safety. What are the dangers? For example, unplug the stove while the caregiver is gone.

"You can't always be there for everything every minute."

Bonnie and Jenn ask how they're addressing the issue of driving. Driving is a sign of freedom, and it's hard to give up.

A mother announces, "I don't have any problems." Shaking her head, her daughter rolls her eyes as Mom continues, "Nobody's going to make me stop driving!"

As everyone laughs with her, a client chimes in, "When you've come home and the car is damaged, that's a sign."

When this latest chorus of chuckles ends, Bonnie shifts gears.

"What will it be like when you can't drive? Can you agree on it? What are the signs to evaluate when you can't drive? You need to talk about those now."

A sign might be an increased number of parking lot accidents that are "someone else's fault." She explains that it's much harder for men to give up driving because it's such a huge part of who they are. Families have to find alternatives to get them where they want or need to go. *(See more on driving on page 138.)*

That's definitely some fuel for the drive home ...

32

The following week, clients and caregivers return for another session, this time focusing on the topic of stress. Facilitator Bonnie offers several suggestions:

▶ *Relax by sitting on the porch.*

▶ *Call someone who will just listen. "Just being heard is important."*

▶ *Having a pet is a great stress reliever.*

▶ *Escape from the reality of the moment by daydreaming.*

▶ *What you're feeling is normal, "part of caregiving, part of being human." The sensation of being overwhelmed — not getting enough sleep, depression, health problems, inability to concentrate — leads to a "big ball of stress."*

▶ *Anger or blaming yourself makes stress worse.*

▶ *Remove yourself from the source of stress by getting out and exercising in fresh air.*

▶ *Give the brain and body a rest.*

▶ *It doesn't take long to relax if you really want to. Breathe out fear, anxiousness and not knowing. Breathe in quiet and peace. Let the positive fill you because you can go to it any time you want.*

After a brief discussion, they break into two groups: the clients stay with Jenn and the caregivers go with Bonnie.

Facilitator Jenn asks the clients for ways to help them remember everyday tasks ...

"Inefficiency causes stress."

One puts his keys and wallet in the same place all the time. He uses a pill organizer.

"(My own system) may not be as good as hers, but it's my way."

Storing phone numbers in the phone helps.

It's frustrating because one man forgets where he leaves things.

"I'm happy when I find things. One star for me!"

One is trying to organize a regular routine.

A daily schedule helps another so he can learn what to expect.

Jenn encourages them to interact more by asking, "What do you do for enjoyment?"

"I read books. I wasn't a reader. I am now. I read everything."

"I ought to get into reading."

"I should have a dog. That's what I miss."

Another golfs every day.

33

"I never dreamed I'd be satisfied not doing much."

"I'm doing nothing."

"If I'm not busy, I start thinking, and that's not always good."

Soon it turns into a sharing of mutual frustrations of losing not only their memory, but their independence ...

A neighbor tells her to go no further than the corner on her walk.

"If I didn't have (my wife), I'd have a nervous breakdown."

Her daughter calls every day and asks if she's taken her medicine. "She doesn't trust me when I say yes. I have to go get them."

"I rely on (my wife) way too much. I may be in trouble someday."

It's a problem and blessing when his wife takes care of everything.

"You have to be honest with yourself."

"If I have a problem, I can contact somebody."

Her children call every day, and she has wonderful neighbors.

"Things I used to do automatically, things are different now."

A former sales representative drove thousands of miles and now can't drive by himself. "It's a hard adjustment."

One says his sister told him he couldn't burn a candle, not even a little one.

Another reminds him, "They're looking out for you ..."

Jenn asks if they become stressed at their caregivers.

One husband volunteers, "I don't have stress. I give her stress."

Some say their spouses tell them what to do all the time.

"My wife is a workaholic and would rather be at work than with me," one man says.

"I wish I could get her to do something around the house."

"I'm sad. She's retired and out volunteering. I think she wants to divorce me." He laughs.

"You're alone," one man explains. "It's frustrating to me. It gets frustrating. I try to talk to her sometimes, like she doesn't hear me. I can't watch football, but she can watch soap operas. I go rake leaves."

"I tell the truth," says another.

"There are times when I can't cope with it," one admits.

Some everyday adjustments are much easier than others

Dave's cardiac arrest and loss of oxygen to the brain several years ago introduced Dave and Sally to the world of dementia and memory loss. While he may have lost his short-term memory, he hasn't misplaced his life-long sense of humor.

"I've always been such a superior person that it was hard for her to tell" that he had memory loss.

Smiling, Sally says, "No ego at all." She recounts how he answered a hospital nurse when she asked how he got there. "Well, 72 years ago, my mother and father got together, and out I popped."

This long-time salesman suffered cardiac arrest at home and the lack of oxygen contributed to the dementia and forgetfulness he experiences today. Thankfully, Sally says, it's consistent and will likely not worsen as he's still able to care for himself.

"I didn't know I had a heart attack. It was a silent one," he says. "I just went on with my normal life."

Well, that's not the whole story. Sally explains that he was in rehabilitation for two months at a nursing home. She noticed the memory changes immediately, and he was tested for Alzheimer's.

He laughs. "I don't remember that. I've got another problem, loss of memory."

"I was so lucky," she remembers. "He didn't want to drive again. That was very fortunate."

After a bout of depression, the doctor wanted to add a new medication to his regimen. Sally objected because of the volume he was already taking. Instead, Dave opted for one martini at the same time every day, and she reports that he's actually done better. Because of diabetes, he's also on a strict dietary schedule.

"I decided I'd have one drink a day," Dave says, "and I look forward to it. It's enough to keep me happy."

When the visitor asks if he thinks he has a memory problem, he says, "I think it's getting better. I remember my wife and when we got married. I remember my kids' names.

"I used to know how much we had in the bank account until I turned it over to her." Everyone laughs. "The sheriff hasn't knocked on the door, so she's doing all right."

In her own words

What worries Delores most about having Alzheimer's?

"It drives me crazy. That's about it. It drives you crazy. I'd like to go and drive and get out. Now I gotta wait for somebody always. It just makes me mad. Not that it's going to do any good."

Does she hold in the anger?

"I guess. It just drives me nuts." Tears fill her eyes. "Just goofy. There are things I want to do that I can't go out and do. That's my car, and I haven't driven it for a year and a half. If I have to put it up a tree, I'll drive it. They tell me I'm not going to, but I'm going to. It's mine. It's in my name. I bought it. That makes it mine, doesn't it?"

The visitor nods in sympathy.

What does Delores want people to know about Alzheimer's?

"I don't talk to anybody about it. There's nobody. Who would you talk to about it?"

What would she tell someone about what she's going through?

"I don't know. Blow your head off, I guess. It's just frustrating, you know."

What does she want her family to understand?

"I don't know. Nothing, I guess. They're not going to change. I'm going to change. It's so confining. I'm used to getting up and going. I always used to. I had my car."

Living in this house for more than 60 years, she used to work in housekeeping at a nursing home and talked to residents often.

"It's frustrating."

Her advice to other families?

"Try to stay sane."

Her daughter, Donna, joins her at the kitchen table. Donna talks about the challenge of having both parents with Alzheimer's. Does she worry about the same fate? "At this point, I don't really want to know. I'm dealing with this right now."

Delores looks up from the table and announces, "We'll all get a big bullet and shoot ourselves."

Everyone laughs. Donna suggests another option.

"We'll get a cannon and all just stand in front it."

Delores nods and grins.

Caregivers say...

In our daily lives, we are inundated with so much information in person and via the media that we have to filter it and decide what's important to us at this moment. It's often only when someone we know has a certain condition that we start to tune in to feed a hunger to learn more. And then we realize other friends and family have or are experiencing the same thing. Eerie, isn't it?

What did you know about Alzheimer's, dementia or memory loss before this person was diagnosed?

▸ Not much

▸ General information

▸ A lot

▸ No family history

▸ Three generations with it

▸ Worked in adult day care

▸ Worked in Alzheimer's unit

▸ Employed as a nurse

▸ His mother and sister had it

▸ Caseworker for seniors

▸ Just what was in the media

▸ Her aunt and grandma had it

▸ More than most people

▸ Her father had it

▸ Read about it

▸ I worked as a CNA before, so I knew quite a bit. *Shallen, 25, grandmother, Alzheimer's*

▸ I thought I knew a lot as I took care of Alzheimer's patients in a nursing home. Only I saw them when it was close to the last stages. I've learned a lot with Mom. *Jenny, 56, mother, Alzheimer's*

▸ Not a lot, although I suppose my maternal grandfather had it, but then no one really had a name for it. *Norma, 81, mother, Alzheimer's, died 11 years after diagnosed; sister, Alzheimer's, died 6 years after diagnosed*

"I didn't know much except that it was a long-term disease."
Leora, 72, husband, Alzheimer's

▸ Little. Our son gave the legal aspect information of a five-part program. *Robert, 77, wife, Alzheimer's*

▸ I have an uncle who had it so my aunt kept me informed. *Maxine, 77, husband, Alzheimer's*

▸ I had served on the board of the local Alzheimer's chapter. *John, 59, mother, Alzheimer's*

▸ Nothing. You heard about memory loss, but I guess you didn't pay attention as you should have. *Robert, 79, wife, Alzheimer's, died 6 years after diagnosed*

▸ Lots and I had already joined a private list online. *Marlene, 68, husband, dementia/Alzheimer's*

▸ I am a nurse and worked with geriatrics in the acute and home setting. *Kim, 34, grandmother, died 5 years after diagnosed*

▸ Some. His father had recently died of Alzheimer's, but my husband was the one most involved there. *June, 66, husband, early onset Alzheimer's*

▸ I have worked with hospice and had many dementia patients. *Martha, 71, husband, cognitive decline*

▸ My grandmother had geriatric Alzheimer's, but I knew nothing about early onset. *Vicky, 54, husband, early onset Alzheimer's, died 5 years after diagnosed*

▸ I studied psychology in college and had to learn specific information about kinds of memory loss. *Marcy, 76, husband, memory loss due to massive stroke*

▸ Very little, just that people lose their memories slowly. *Jody, 47, mother, early onset Alzheimer's*

▸ Quite a lot. I am an RN and have had many patients with the disease. *Kevin, 45, mother, Alzheimer's*

▸ That it was terminal, of long duration, unpleasant. *Catherine, 85, husband, Alzheimer's and Lewy Body*

"My vision of Alzheimer's was something exclusive to old people." Andrew, 25, father, frontal lobe dementia, diagnosed at age 51

"Step on toes if you have to ... they'll get over it"

When her mother, Delores, was diagnosed with Alzheimer's, Donna recalls, it followed a long period of forgetting names, repeating questions and forgetting to write down check amounts.

Then she got the same news about her father a year later. She says he should have been diagnosed earlier but getting him to see a doctor was a struggle. She had to use renewing his driver's license as blackmail.

The daughter realized that her dad was having problems and suddenly asking directions while driving. He'd get mad and blame everything wrong on everybody else. He was mad that he couldn't fix Delores. They had him tested and started him on anti-depressants. He has trouble with speech patterns and forgets stuff, but she constantly repeats herself.

"I think we all took it in stride. It's part of life. Some people have it, some people don't ..." As one of five adult children, Donna changed jobs and took a third-shift position so she could help them during the day. They rely on Meals on Wheels for most of their lunches and dinners, mostly because they like them.

When they go out to eat, Delores presses the word "ice" on the self-serve soda machine and can't understand why it doesn't dispense ice. She usually orders what another person selects. When asked about salad dressing, Donna lets her know she likes them all. "I think she doesn't want to make a mistake."

Donna says it's harder on everyone during bad weather.

"She's used to getting out. During the winter, they were here looking at each other 24/7. You get tired of looking at someone." She laughs. Her mother said one snowy day that it was days like this when she was cooped up with the kids when they were little that she wrote a relative, "I need to get out or I'll kill somebody." Donna took her out the next day.

Her parents fell on their 59th anniversary and ended up in emergency room. Though the details have changed with each re-telling, Delores was helping him off the couch, and they both fell.

Donna has noticed an odd pattern in how her mother interprets time. Everything seems to happen in three-week intervals, i.e., the dog hasn't eaten anything in three weeks or she's been broke for three weeks.

"Loss of independence, that's killing her more than anything."

Delores kept running out of cash but actually misplaced it. Donna learned to give her less money over time and allocate it in small bills to make it look like more.

"She's dealing with it as a power struggle, and what she can control is the food in her mouth." Delores is also diabetic and getting her to eat properly has been frustrating for everyone. If they don't watch her closely, she'll eat just bread. Trying to explain to her that a glass of orange juice is not a meal is fruitless. Whatever she's given, she'll eat only half to rebel. They've explained to her that she'll end up in the hospital or a nursing home, and they won't release her if she's not getting proper nutrition.

The adult children plan to keep them at home as long as possible, she explains. A sister who recently retired has helped considerably. "As Mom says, Dad's a step behind her."

What has she learned so far to share with other families?

"You need to be prepared, patient and get their affairs in order. People say, 'I've got time, I've got time,' but things go quickly." Delores has some bad days when she forgets to check her blood sugar. A good day for her dad is when he can write his name.

"You need to take time off because it wears on you. Stay connected with your own family. They understand. They're patient."

Her husband's grandmother had dementia, so he understands. It's best to get them diagnosed ASAP. "Step on toes if you have to. They'll get over it. Once things are forgotten, you can't retrieve them."

The good thing about both parents having Alzheimer's is that she can tell each of them that the other needs something. She talked to the pharmacist regularly to see if they were getting medications properly. Delores told her one day, "Oh yeah, they gave it to me but forgot to charge me for it." Donna didn't buy that excuse. Now she picks up everything herself. "Hopefully I'll never get pulled over because I've got medications for two different people." She laughs.

She calls every night after the news to make sure they've taken their medicine. She's learned to keep them on the phone until she's sure they've completed this task.

Even when she's taken her mom out for the day, Delores tells people she hasn't been out in weeks, because she can't remember. Donna's trying to get other relatives and friends involved, but she's discovered that people say they're going to do something but don't.

Keep up a regular routine

Sue recalls:"I kept things as calm as possible in the house, a similar routine every day, because any little unusual thing could get her nervous. I was always able to keep her from having any anger outburst by self-talking myself, 'Stay calm. Don't let it upset you. Remember, she's got an illness.' That way I didn't get frustrated."

Daughter discovers special relationship

June says, "My daughter tells me how she's changed her viewpoint. She used to be so angry and upset that her children would never know their grandpa. But when she watches grandpa and her two and a half year old play by the hour, she now realizes that her kids will know grandpa in a way very few children do. My husband and grandson are content with each other and the rest of the world isn't there! They are very close. Such a special relationship!"

"Confusing disease! He has good days, then bad days. He remembers things, then forgets everything."
Pat, 66, husband, Alzheimer's

"You *never, never* argue"

Bonnie has heard and seen it all during her decade as an education specialist at the Alzheimer's Association.

"One thing I have found interesting is that many caregivers don't define themselves as that," she explains. "We really had a struggle getting people, when we offered a caregivers class, for them to realize they're a caregiver. They're *just* the spouse or child who's taking care of the person, but they don't see it much differently than being a parent who's a caregiver. They don't see it in that terminology. Sometimes they don't identify themselves as that so they can reach out to get help. I've noticed that many of them don't realize (what we have available)."

41

This chapter tried to put together an early-stage support group for nearly five years before enough people signed up. Families tend to not come in as much in the beginning, Bonnie says.

What is the one great truth that families must accept?

"You *never, never* argue with a person with dementia. It's a challenge, but you can do it. The more support you have and the more you know, the easier it will be.

"The stigma is less, but it's still out there. What I know is on personal levels, social circles will stop calling and avoid people. It's kind of like what happens in a divorce. What do they think it is, contagious? It's similar, but it's different. Most social circles are the same age, and it's kind of 'if it can happen to you, it can happen to me.' When we don't know how to do something or understand, we avoid it. The person who may have once been the life of the party now sits there saying nothing," she says.

"What we see a lot of is denial. We see that in the families, whether it's the spouse or the grown kids; it's about fear. 'If I don't believe it, I don't have to deal with it. If I don't believe it, it's not going to happen. If I don't believe it, maybe the doctor was wrong, and life will go back to the way it was.' Unscientifically, I see it more among the adult children, more in the males than the females.

"Just from my observations, and I don't have any hard numbers, it's more difficult for men to deal with something where there is not a concrete, 10-step checklist. 'Here's what you need to do, and you will have fixed it for Mom and Dad.' The nebulous, the grayness of all this, what may work today may not work tomorrow, seems to be more difficult for the males." She hears from many families that daughters and daughters-in-law are more involved.

Research many sources
of information on dementia

It would take many lifetimes to read and absorb the abundance of written material about Alzheimer's, dementia and memory loss. Actually, it would be impossible because new material is created 24/7. Information about these subjects, as life itself, is ever-evolving.

It's important not to rely on only one source when learning more about these complex topics. Ask for details from your physician and his office staff. Study reliable books and magazine articles. Consult the Alzheimer's Association *(www.alz.org)* and other aging-related organizations. Check out the Internet, but remember that some Web sites do not include documentation as to the source of materials.

Listening and talking about issues related to these conditions also provide valuable learning experiences. We can garner much by opening our ears and minds to what other families have confronted through various stages.

When hearing this type of diagnosis, we can often remember other individuals who had similar experiences. See if they're willing to share the highs and lows as you begin your own journey. You'd be surprised at how willing they may be to help others with their first-hand knowledge.

It could also help them in *their* healing process.

"I have a master's degree in nursing and taught at a community college. I thought I knew a lot."
Sandy, 61, husband, Alzheimer's and vascular dementia

Professionals say...

While tending to the needs of many dementia and memory loss patients, professional caregivers have discovered the value of a variety of resources for families to help them cope.

43

How can families best educate themselves?

▸ Read, attend support groups, check the Internet. *Kalah, 48, social service assistant, four months*

▸ Know what to expect and how to handle their behavior. *Pam, 44, LPN, 25 years*

▸ Support groups, books, videos. *Dave, 40, executive director, 2 years*

▸ Attend seminars, talk to other caregivers, read books, etc. *Cindy, 53, nurse, 34 years*

▸ Work or volunteer time with afflicted persons. *Marge, 50, nursing home administrator, 24 years*

▸ Research the disease, attend meetings, etc. *Sherry, 27, trainer, 2 years*

▸ Contact the Alzheimer's Association, attend all conferences, computer. *Sharon, 55, nurse aide/driver, 15 years*

▸ Books, DVDs, attend conferences, talk to others. Support groups, too. *Connie, 57, psychotherapist*

▸ Ask questions, research and educate themselves as much as possible. *Michelle, 48, CNA, 30 years*

▸ Get as much information that they can get any way they can get it. *Gloria, 54, CNA, 18 years*

▸ Keep up on the research and attend self-care groups. *Edi, social worker, 17 years*

▸ Support groups and being involved with the Alzheimer's Association. *Mary, 37, hospital social worker, 11 years*

▸ Read, visit a unit, volunteer. *Trudy, 57, director of nursing, 30 years*

Professionals say...

The professionals who work with dementia and memory loss patients every day in a variety of settings each bring unique life experiences to the job. Here are some examples.

What background prepared you for this field?

▸ I helped care for my great-grandmother at home until she passed. *Latoya, 27, CNA, 2 years*

▸ Bachelor of arts degree in psychology, interest in the field. *Kalah, 48, social service assistant, four months*

▸ I love to work with the elderly. *Pam, 44, LPN, 25 years*

▸ Nursing, job experience, home care, caregiving, seminars. *Cindy, 53, nurse, 34 years*

▸ Three years at a senior living center. *Sherry, 27, trainer, 2 years*

▸ Adult day care since 1992. *Ronni, R.N, 49, 28 years*

▸ Certification and working on hospital floor. *Sharon, 55, nurse aide/driver, 15 years*

▸ Bachelor of science degree in psychology, MSW, LCSW, 29 years experience. *Connie, 57, psychotherapist*

▸ Home care with elderly. *Michelle, 48, CNA, 30 years*

▸ Taking care of people in their homes. *Gloria, 54, CNA, 18 years*

▸ Work on Alzheimer's unit. *Susan, 38, R.N., 12 years*

▸ Attended Alzheimer's conference for the past six years. *Edi, social worker, 17 years*

▸ Nursing home experience. *Trudy, 57, director of nursing, 30 years*

▸ Working in long-term care and skilled care facilities. *Vicki, 56, R.N., 35 years*

▸ Sheltered care with dementia and Alzheimer's residents. *Susan, 58, LPN*

▸ Art therapy and behavioral science, social work. *Michelle, 38, 11 years*

Caregivers say...

It seems like the medical community comes up with a new disease or condition every week. When we see someone exhibit certain symptoms or behaviors, we often ask ourselves, *"I wonder if ..."* However, when it comes to Alzheimer's, we make jokes about having "Old-Timers Disease" because we're all forgetful at times. Yet, when it comes to someone we love, our gut reaction is, *"Nah, it can't be ..."* though the possibility lurks uncomfortably within us.

45

With the change in behavior, what did you first believe was occurring? When did you think it could be Alzheimer's, memory loss or dementia?

- A stroke
- TIA's
- History of Alzheimer's in family
- Severe depression
- Alcoholism

- Hearing loss
- Dementia
- Just aging
- Absentmindedness
- Sleeping disorder

- We thought that it might have been dementia, but we also thought her medicine played a role. Finally, a neurologist diagnosed her. *Shallen, 25, grandmother, Alzheimer's*

- I really didn't know or maybe didn't want to accept it. *Jolene, 66, mother, dementia, died 5 years after diagnosed*

- I was told by the physician after his stroke that Alzheimer's might occur, and it has. *Christl, 55, father, stroke and Alzheimer's*

"I thought at first he had a small stroke, then thought he was worked up due to worry about treatments he was to have for prostate cancer."
Pat, 66, husband, Alzheimer's

46

▸ I knew what it was after an episode of Dad getting lost and very emotional. At that time, we'd just moved back home, so I hadn't seen him much to observe more symptoms. *Ann, 49, mother, vascular dementia, died; father, Alzheimer's, died*

▸ After getting hearing aids, we saw improvement, then erratic behavior (confusion) when out of her environment. *Cathi, 58, mother, dementia*

▸ I recognized it could be Alzheimer's long before her doctor. I started going to the doctor with her. She would tell him everything was okay. I had to tell him what was going on. *Jenny, 56, mother, Alzheimer's*

▸ I was afraid of dementia. I retired and knew some changes were occurring. *Leora, 72, husband, Alzheimer's*

▸ I suspected with my sister when she lost her way to my home. She lived 100 miles away and had traveled the road for 50 years. She lost interest in eating and had trouble with keeping her checkbook. Three years earlier she was running a business. *Norma, 81, mother, Alzheimer's, died 11 years after diagnosed; sister, Alzheimer's, died 6 years after diagnosed*

▸ When it was diagnosed. *Phil, 69, mother, dementia*

▸ It was so gradual. I had seven children to care for and working out of the home. When something went wrong, I made adjustments. *Roseann, 72, husband, dementia, died 10 years after diagnosed*

▸ At first, I thought he just wasn't paying attention. I first thought Alzheimer's when he totally forgot an important family tradition. *June, 66, husband, early onset Alzheimer's*

▸ I began doing research and suspected my husband had Alzheimer's. He would read me the movie schedule over and over and over again. The same with the obituaries, and he would go to the fridge and list me the contents. *Marlene, 68, husband, dementia/Alzheimer's*

"I was confused until she got fired from her job. After that you start thinking." David, 69, wife, Alzheimer's

- Initially I thought she was being careless. The likelihood of Alzheimer's arose quickly. *Elizabeth, 47, mother, Alzheimer's*

- Alzheimer's never crossed my mind due to my dad's young age. *Andrew, 25, father, frontal lobe dementia, diagnosed at age 51*

- We weren't sure if it was Alzheimer's or alcoholism. *Kim, 34, grandmother, died 5 years after diagnosed*

- When coronary bypass surgery led to a stroke and coma in 1997, his memory came back slowly and incompletely. *Marcy, 76, husband, memory loss due to massive stroke*

- When she would mistake me for her sister. *Sally, 57, mother, Alzheimer's, died 3 years after diagnosed*

- We were both in denial. *Bill, 78, wife, Alzheimer's, died 4 years after diagnosed*

- Dad sought a diagnosis very early due to family history, and he is a slight hypochondriac. *Mary, 38, father, Alzheimer's*

- At first dementia. Within 12 months Alzheimer's. *J, grandmother, Alzheimer's*

- During a test given by a doctor in 2001, he couldn't tell the season, where he was, where he was born, but he was functioning normally otherwise. *Catherine, 85, husband, Alzheimer's and Lewy Body*

- I was pretty sure of the signs and behavior after I had experienced the disease with my mother and sister. *Norma, 81, husband, Alzheimer's*

- I prayed it wasn't Alzheimer's, but her mom and sister had Alzheimer's, so I was pretty sure it was. *MM, 46, mother, Alzheimer's, died 5 years after diagnosed*

- I thought she was drinking too much beer. She acted the same way without beer. Mainly, the loss of interest in life. *Gayle, 59, mother, Alzheimer's, died 5 years after diagnosed*

"Not paying attention. Her doctor hospitalized her and called me." Ann, 63, aunt, Alzheimer's, died 6 years after diagnosed

"No one believed me"

The words read like a broken record, *"No one believed me ..."*

Many caregivers have described the frustration and pain of enduring weeks, months or even years of knowing *something* was not right with their loved one ... episodes of forgetfulness, odd behavior, lack of personal grooming, confusion and other symptoms of dementia or memory loss.

But no one believed them.

Spouses of individuals with Alzheimer's or related conditions may see the day-to-day progression or deterioration. Or the adult child who keeps in frequent contact with a parent may notice curious or unusual behavior. They mention it to others, who may not notice any alarming changes because they don't see the parent as often or only talk on the phone ... during a 15-minute conversation.

Even doctors have discounted a loved one's concern because the patient seems just fine ... during a 15-minute office visit.

The caregiver sees it 24/7, yet the afflicted individual often puts on an award-winning performance for everyone else ... during a 15-minute encounter.

There are countless heartbreaking accounts of caregivers who were accused of lying, exaggerating, being overbearing, stealing, causing trouble or being the ones who have "the" problem. One woman recalls how her adult daughter berated her mercilessly over the phone for even suggesting that her father had Alzheimer's ... *"Nothing's wrong with Dad!* You've *got the problem!"* The caregiver succumbed to tears under the attack ... and again when recounting the brutal exchange.

Yes, the world will always play host to hypochondriacs and individuals who constantly crave attention, and people who try to take advantage of another's illness or misfortune. However, there are many who deny a situation like dementia or memory loss, either in silence or by loudly proclaiming their refusal to believe.

Many families' bonds are at risk of being eroded or severed in addressing an Alzheimer's diagnosis. Sad stories are prevalent of siblings who became estranged during the decision-making process of caring for a parent. Sadder yet are the tales of those adult children who refuse to make amends even long after the parent passes away.

Ask yourself: *Is denial easier than facing a painful truth?*
That's why they call it denial.

Though certainly not easy to accept, maladies such as cancer or heart disease can be more readily grasped as medical testing and treatment is a more exact science. With dementia or memory loss, it's harder to list a definitive cause and often is not 100 percent conclusive until an autopsy ... obviously a tragic after-the-fact revelation. However, the medical community has made tremendous strides in recent years in diagnosing Alzheimer's and related conditions.

49

Admittedly, dementia and memory loss are difficult to understand, particularly since everyone responds and progresses differently. In addition, what we cannot see, what is hidden within our brains, is often viewed with skepticism when someone we love looks the same. As noted previously, adult children often have a more difficult time accepting these conditions, especially if they're not in daily or weekly contact with the parents.

That's another reason why early diagnosis is critical, not only for the individual's well-being, but to allow family and friends to address immediate and future needs of everyone affected. While explaining details with those who had been in denial:

▸ *Decide what size and setting is best to share this information, whether as a large group, a half-dozen or individually. You should know what will work best, given the circumstances, and whether someone is more likely to respond with grief, anger and myriad emotions ... or if they need to be around loved ones or alone.*

▸ *Share pertinent details that highlight the facts upon which the physician based the diagnosis. Be prepared to discuss options and opportunities for medication(s) the doctor recommends.*

▸ *Avoid creating a stage for confrontation and accusations. Don't expect or request that decisions be made immediately. Let the news soak in. Create a priority list that best serves the needs of the loved one with dementia or memory loss, one that includes their input if they're still able to contribute to their caregiving plans.*

Remember to listen to family members' reactions and not be afraid to share yours. Pay attention, as useful suggestions and offers of assistance may be expressed.

It may be difficult, but be gracious if they apologize for not believing you sooner. This is *not* a time for, *"I told you so."*

"She'd mask it and we'd say never mind"

50

Ask Char and Jim about Alzheimer's and dementia. They have accumulated too much first-hand knowledge in caring for both of their mothers.

Here's their first encounter with Alzheimer's.

Jim noticed that his mother was exhibiting signs of forgetfulness and paying bills twice or not at all, which was uncharacteristic of a woman who had always been meticulous about paperwork. After his brother shared his experiences of coping with an in-law with Alzheimer's, Jim's suspicions mounted.

"Dad just let her do what she wanted. He was in denial for several years, which is not all that unusual response for his generation. Who would want to admit that? He acted like she'd snap out of it and change her attitude, like a sickness she'd get over. He said, 'You just wait until you get old and you'll find out ...' " They took him to a couple of Alzheimer's Association seminars to try to educate him on the disease and how it would progress and worsen. It took a long time to convince him, Jim says.

"Her defense mechanisms were very good. We'd ask a question, and she'd answer with a question and say anything but answer your question." She'd go to the store, not return for hours and make excuses about why she was late. They later heard that she had been wandering in the parking lot looking for her car.

"She had a lot of pride, and she would not admit she didn't know something. She was an intelligent person. She would mask it, and we'd say 'never mind.' "

They also discovered a growing mass of mail. "She wasn't able to sift through this and make decisions," Char says. The situation worsened when she had taken some money and invested it without telling the rest of the family. These were more than "senior moments."

Jim says, "It took more than a year to sift through all the paperwork, stop the mailings and sales calls, and organize all the bills. She was from the Depression era and kept everything for decades. Papers were piled up and stuffed in drawers. You'd find a utility bill from this month and right next to it would be something from 1950 or 1970."

The process of sifting through bills, legal papers, financial records, and health matters is an important first step before getting durable power of attorney for property and health.

As she continued "losing that grasp on day-to-day living," they discovered spoiled food and mismatched clothes. Luckily, she said she wanted to give up cooking and live elsewhere, so this was the opportunity to move them to a seniors facility. The family was relieved.

However, within a few months, she was obviously confused and disoriented as she was found roaming at night, Jim says. She thought she was still cooking but wasn't. She was critical of his dad, everything and everyone as she continued to fall further out of touch with reality. Jim's dad attempted to be her caregiver, but he didn't know what to do because they couldn't communicate. Jim says they all quickly learned that they could not talk rationally with an Alzheimer's patient.

"He had to live with her 24 hours a day, and he said, 'You don't know what it's like, living all day long with somebody you can't carry on a conversation with.' It drove him crazy, day after day, week after week, and that would have an effect on anybody, especially somebody you've been living with for 50 years. You can't accept that they're losing their mind," Jim says. "We could remain a little more objective by not being there all day."

They soon moved her into an assisted living facility and his dad into a studio apartment, an arrangement that benefitted her while allowing him some independence. However, she soon slipped out of the facility and one time, fell down in a nearby field. A couple of times she said she had to get back home. When asked where home was, she stated that it was the farm where she had lived as a child.

"She was strong-willed and stubborn, and nobody was keeping her in there," Jim remembers. Finally, she required medication to calm and keep her from wandering.

They found attending Alzheimer's Association meetings particularly helpful as they could stay ahead of what would likely happen next. Jim learned to rationalize that this was the disease, not his mother.

Eventually, she fell, broke her hip and was hospitalized. She participated in some physical therapy and used a walker though she became more dependent on a wheelchair.

"Her mind wouldn't tell her body to move," Jim says. They learned that it's not unusual for Alzheimer's patients to forget the therapy learned for walking and even standing.

Jim recalls one Christmas when they gave her gift certificates and other items, and she claimed she didn't get anything.

"So, we went on a treasure hunt to look for the gift certificates that she had unknowingly stuffed in her dresser drawer." His advice? "Don't give them anything valuable because they have a way of hiding things, and you'll never find them."

As a few years passed, her medical condition deteriorated. She lost her ability to communication and make eye contact. Jim recalls when she forgot how to swallow as memory of that reflex was disconnected in her brain. She eventually contracted pneumonia and passed away.

During all this, Jim says he witnessed many other families go through more difficult circumstances and some even leave a patient in a nursing home and never visit again. He admits that it was almost a relief when his mother died after being bedridden for months. He also learned that people think their situations are completely different, but most families confront similar issues. That's why it's important to ask for help from the Alzheimer's Association and others who have endured these difficult times.

"It's like cancer. You hardly know a family that hasn't been affected by cancer. It's the same with Alzheimer's. It's not just getting old and forgetful. It's the bizarre stuff, too. You may know it in your heart that she's slipping, but in your head, you can talk yourself out of it. You deny reality. (Families) don't know how to cope, but sometimes they don't want advice."

High-profile patients like Ronald Reagan and Charleston Heston have helped promote awareness.

"You have to accept the cycle of life and getting older. You deal with it and hang on to the good times," he says. "It's the disease talking, but it's hard not to take it personally."

Professionals say...

Individuals in the healthcare field who care for dementia and memory loss patients select this focus for a variety of personal or professional reasons.

Why have you devoted yourself to caring for individuals with Alzheimer's?

53

▸ It's a sad situation and sometimes we can forget that the clients once lived a normal life just as we do. *Latoya, 27, CNA, 2 years*

▸ I'm very interested in the disease and how to best help them. *Kalah, 48, social service assistant, four months*

▸ To give people dignity. My grandmother and father had the disease. *Dave, 40, executive director, 2 years*

▸ I seem to connect with them. I've always loved the geriatric population. It's very rewarding and fulfilling. *Cindy, 53, nurse, 34 years*

▸ Because the disease has so many negative connotations. *Marge, 50, nursing home administrator, 24 years*

▸ I want to educate myself though hands-on experience. I have grown emotionally attached and have a strong compassion for the clients I encounter every day. I enjoy what I'm doing. *Sherry, 27, trainer, 2 years*

▸ The satisfaction from helping the families care for their loved ones. *Ronni, R.N, 49, 28 years*

▸ I do home care and enjoy keeping people from going to skilled care facilities as long as possible. *Michelle, 48, CNA, 30 years*

▸ Now my husband has some of the problems that a person with Alzheimer's has. *Gloria, 54, CNA, 18 years*

▸ I have to. I work mainly with adults. Dad has Alzheimer's. *Karen, 46, developmental technician, 20 years*

▸ My grandmother and beloved mother-in-law had Alzheimer's. *Susan, 58, LPN*

▸ I love our residents. It's like with children, the experiences change every day. They teach us a lot. It's a reward. A reason for living is giving. *Trudy, 57, director of nursing, 30 years*

What do you feel your role is?

▶ To help clients live with dignity and without shame. *Latoya, 27, CNA, 2 years*

▶ To advocate for good quality care for our seniors, to be a good friend/person for them to be able to rely on. *Kalah, 48, social service assistant, four months*

▶ Making their last days enjoyable. *Pam, 44, LPN, 25 years*

▶ Give all the proper tools and training for staff to provide excellent care. *Dave, 40, executive director, 2 years*

▶ Patient and family support. Family education. Keeping patients safe, meeting their needs. *Cindy, 53, nurse, 34 years*

▶ Setting the mood for staff and being a source of relief for families, a sounding board of sorts. *Marge, 50, nursing home administrator, 24 years*

▶ Be there for the patients and try to understand what they are going through. *Sherry, 27, trainer, 2 years*

▶ Help families to maintain patients in their own environment for as long as they're able. *Ronni, R.N, 49, 28 years*

▶ To help reduce family members' stress and help patients enjoy the remainder of their years. *Sharon, 55, nurse aide/driver, 15 years*

▶ To help families reach a healthy adjustment and improve the quality of relationships. *Connie, 57, psychotherapist*

▶ Be supportive, help educate, teach how to relate to patients with Alzheimer's or dementia. *Michelle, 48, CNA, 30 years*

▶ Friend, caregiver. *Gloria, 54, CNA, 18 years*

▶ I don't know anymore. I get as frustrated as anyone else. My role? To be the eyes and ears, the memory and to offer the comforting touch. *Karen, 46, developmental technician, 20 years*

▶ Helping them to be as independent as possible. *Debi, 48, trainer, 6 years*

▶ Listening, being there for them, be their friend for the day. Redirecting their behavior when possible. *Vicki, 56, R.N., 35 years*

▶ Caregiver for both family and resident. Educator, giving hope to families, peace and security to resident. *Susan, 58, LPN*

Caregivers say...

Many people try to prepare themselves to hear bad news. It's supposed to make the blow easier to absorb. Everybody responds differently to hearing the diagnosis of Alzheimer's, memory loss or dementia. That's what confuses us when someone doesn't respond the same way we do. Be aware that everyone absorbs, copes and behaves differently, so don't automatically label someone else as uncaring or insincere. Some people prefer to react privately. Let them, yet be there if they need you.

55

What was your reaction to this person being diagnosed?

▸ Shocked

▸ Not surprised

▸ Sad

▸ Worried about his quality of life

▸ Heartbroken

▸ Depressed

▸ Very surprised

▸ Sorrow

▸ Confirmed suspicions

▸ Relief

▸ Anger

▸ Loneliness

▸ Fear of the future

▸ Acceptance

▸ Mourning

▸ Grief

▸ Crushed

▸ Determined to care for her

▸ Relief that medication was available

▸ Had the need to protect her

▸ Concerned

▸ Denial

"We wanted a second opinion because we did not believe the doctor." Shallen, 25, grandmother, Alzheimer's

56

- Satisfaction because now we knew what we were dealing with. *Laurie, 47, father, dementia*

- We grew into it as my father-in-law was ill, and my mother-in-law stayed with us. *John, 67, mother-in-law, Alzheimer's*

- Wanting her to be safe and well-cared for and knowing she could no longer live alone. *Jolene, 66, mother, dementia, died 5 years after diagnosed*

- Feeling that we needed to get my siblings to understand since none of them have a health care background. *Ann, 49, mother, vascular dementia, died; father, Alzheimer's, died*

- I was surprised when the doctor said he shouldn't be left alone. I didn't realize how dangerous it was if something happens. He wouldn't know how to call for help. *Leora, 72, husband, Alzheimer's*

- With Mother, it was hard, but she was older. I adjusted, but with my younger sister, I had a hard time at first. She was not there for me to confide in anymore. We used to finish each other's thoughts. Now I have no one to do that with me. *Norma, 81, mother, Alzheimer's, died 11 years after diagnosed; sister, Alzheimer's, died 6 years after diagnosed*

- Okay, now let's get him on some kind of medication to try to retain as much memory as possible for as long as possible. *Nettie, 51, father, Alzheimer's*

- It helped me realize what the problem was and that he had to be cared for and I needed to learn how. With working, taking care of our family and him, it was a load. *Roseann, 72, husband, dementia, died 10 years after diagnosed*

- I knew he had dementia, but I hated to hear the word Alzheimer's. I have great faith and believe God only gives you what you can handle. *Maxine, 77, husband, Alzheimer's*

- Depressed. How could this be happening to my mother who always had such a good memory? *Darlene, 58, mother, Alzheimer's*

"Scared and depressed. Our life as we knew it was over." Pat, 66, husband, Alzheimer's

▶ Sad. I didn't want to think about it. I cried. I was expecting that's what it was. I knew we had to try hard knowing the battle might be lost. It was worth the effort. *Robert, 79, wife, Alzheimer's, died 6 years after diagnosed*

▶ I was saddened that her future quality of life was clouded by an incurable disease. I worried about *my* own future. Would I suffer the same fate? *Judith, 61, mother, Alzheimer's*

▶ Surprised because of my working with a service organization and being on a committee that chose this focus. *Nancy, 65, mother, Alzheimer's*

▶ Tears, relief to know, glad it wasn't cancer or a tumor, fear of the future, very mixed. *June, 66, husband, early onset Alzheimer's*

▶ Grateful he was alive. Also, there have been no more disagreements because he accepts his memory loss. *Marcy, 76, husband, memory loss due to massive stroke*

▶ We both wanted to doctor it and improve the memory. *Catherine, 85, husband, Alzheimer's and Lewy Body*

▶ It was not a surprise, but it was very hard to have it put into words. That made it too real. *Norma, 81, husband, Alzheimer's*

▶ It was a relief. We finally had an explanation, and I was able to put the pieces of the puzzle (his behavior) together to begin to understand. We knew what we were up against and could move forward with that knowledge. *Andrew, 25, father, frontal lobe dementia, diagnosed 2003 at age 51*

▶ Sadness. She gave direction to make decisions. *J, grandmother, Alzheimer's*

▶ Denial. I couldn't believe God would allow her to get this. *MM, 46, mother, Alzheimer's, died 5 years after diagnosed*

"I was not in shock. I had already expected this. I wanted to help her and be her memory." Jenny, 56, mother, Alzheimer's

Just talking...

(Caregiver and client responses and reactions are in italics.)

Alzheimer's Association facilitator Jenn welcomes everyone back for the third session of the six-week educational and support group program. She opens the conversation by asking for suggestions on remembering dates and where items are placed at home. A monthly calendar for events is often helpful, she says.

A caregiver deadpans, "There are some days I want to cross off completely."

As everyone laughs, Jenn adds, "I have no advice for that."

A variety of thoughts are voiced …

▸ *Habits are hard to break. It's not easy for other people to change their patterns to accommodate yours.*

▸ *Don't hesitate to look at the calendar to remember the day and date.*

▸ *Reading the newspaper helps a lot with remembering dates.*

▸ *Posting phone numbers is helpful, as is caller ID.*

▸ *Be consistent with storing items. Photograph some items to help with memory.*

▸ *Remove clutter. Use sticky notes as reminders to turn things off or something like a whistling teapot to take care of boiling water.*

▸ *Remember that certain tips are not innate to everyone.*

▸ *Allow yourself more time to do things.*

One topic commands the most attention: how caregivers explain things to clients. Caregivers need to understand they may have to detail all the steps in a process, even if it's an automatic response for them and used to be for the individual with dementia or memory loss. They can't take that for granted anymore. Things aren't as simple as they think.

However, the overall message of this portion of the session is that families need to celebrate successes.

After they split into two groups, the caregivers discuss with facilitator Bonnie what's been going in their lives …

One wife finally got her husband to let her fill out the Safe Return bracelet application. She asked him to review it before they brought it in as a way to include him. He understands his own decline. He said, "before too long," that she'll need to keep an eye on him.

His system works for him, even if it's weird to her.

Her mom writes down everything when she takes her medicine.

"I can't get him to change his clothes, take showers and brush his teeth. He won't even clean up to visit the doctor."

The shower issue is a hard, complicated process, Bonnie explains, because spraying water may not be comfortable on the face. Try mouthwash instead of brushing teeth. Ignoring personal hygiene becomes part of the disease, because it's not important to them and likely too complicated. Remember that you may have to break down every step of an action.

"It's like a teenager. Pick your battles," she says.

"I gave the woman at the eye doctor one of the cards explaining he had a memory problem and to please be patient."

"Sometimes it's a control issue. He thinks I'm bossing him around. He forgets. 'You're not my mother!' He wants to be in control. He gets so angry."

B onnie reminds them that their loved ones are losing pieces of themselves, all those things that define who they are. Sometimes they rail at us in frustration.

"We talked this week. He looked at the list of the things to be done and asked if he was getting that bad. It was a clear moment when he asked."

It's all part of the disease, the bad and good days.

Bonnie asks the tough question: have you thought about when you'll have to make decisions for your loved one's future care?

"If something happens to me, our kids know he has to go into a facility. He forgets to eat."

Other health problems will likely kill him before he needs a facility.

The facilitator offers the following thoughts to consider:

▸ *Observe them for pain; don't ask if they're in pain.*

▸ *Non-verbal tells more of what to do than verbal.*

▸ *You have to put on your game face.*

▸ *It's easier to talk about something when you know what's wrong.*

▶ *Reassure them that nobody is avoiding them.*

▶ *Did you see patterns before diagnosis, things that now make sense?*

▶ *Many stock answers cover most Alzheimer's clients' responses to questions. They "fill in the story" around one thought, like embroidering a story around it.*

Bonnie listens as the caregivers continue ...

"He's had friends pull away. Some neighbors became afraid."

"Mom is angry. Nobody will call her. What's wrong?"

"Friends don't call. They're 'too busy.' He doesn't forget they don't call him. He said, 'I don't have any friends.' I call to explain and get them to respond."

Bonnie acknowledges that people pull back out of fear. Would they go out even if the client doesn't say much of anything or nothing at all?

"Dementia really trashes your bridge game," she laments. "People let you down. You're giving up a part of yourself to be immersed in this person. You have to reconnect, though it's hard, to be who *you* are ..."

At the fourth session, communication is the focus. Alzheimer's Association facilitators Jenn and Bonnie encourage them to consider the following tips:

▶ *To get someone's attention, address them by name or apply the soft touch of your hand, if this individual will allow it.*

▶ *Consider the importance of the tone of your voice and non-verbal communication. Attitude and frustration can come out without realizing it.*

▶ *Speak simply, slowly and concisely.*

▶ *Focus on yes and no questions and/or limit their choices in selecting an answer. Avoid "Don't you remember?" questions because those frustrate someone with dementia or memory loss.*

▶ *Don't quiz them, just tell them. It saves their dignity to not quiz them.*

▶ *Accept silence in conversation.*

One client says that she doesn't answer the telephone unless she knows the voice on the answering machine.

A husband turns to his wife in the circle of participants and asks, "I always try to say what I mean, don't I?" She nods. He's visibly relieved.

Another man admits in frustration, "She told me, and I know she told me, but I can't remember."

Everyone nods in sympathy.

Bonnie describes using a notepad as a portable brain.

One client says, "I've got little notes all over the house, but I don't remember where I put them."

61

This time the group smiles in understanding.

And then someone says, "I can't spell or write too well now."

Comprehending that loss is a tough one.

In the breakout session, caregivers and Bonnie share thoughts ...

He kept forgetting and finally decided to take his medicine.

Bonnie explains that they don't believe there is a problem. Caregivers often have to be the bad guy.

Now he can't remember the grandkids' names.

Consider using visual and written cues to help him. Melodies help as do memory boxes.

One wife said her husband has been forgetting her name. The others report they haven't experienced that yet.

It's sad when they can't recognize you. That hurts.

"There was so much I wanted to share at this point in our lives. It really hurts. It's supposed to be the golden years with my best friend." Tears fill her eyes.

"I know there's power in knowledge, but it hurts," another vents.

"I know what's coming."

"It's okay to say, 'why God?' I need to understand. Taking such a vibrant individual, a delightful man ..." She shakes her head in anger.

A husband greeted customers coming into a store.

Savor the pure joy and humor of some situations.

"I couldn't get my husband out of the tub and had to call our son to help get his wet dad out."

That certainly serves as a reality check for an adult child.

Bonnie reminds them that their loved one's brain is slowing down, and that takes a toll on the caregiver, too. It becomes one more thing on our to-prepare-for list.

Talking to the doctor

Visiting the doctor is usually not high on anybody's want-to-do-list, but it's imperative that patient and caregiver take advantage of this precious time to get the answers everyone needs.

To assess the symptoms of dementia and memory loss, your doctor needs all the information he can get to make a proper diagnosis. It's primarily up to the caregiver to come with a prepared list of examples of atypical or worrisome behavior. Caregivers are the ones who usually see the individual every day, and that's why careful observation and notetaking are critical.

Remember to focus on facts, not what you *think* is happening or wrong if you or someone else has not witnessed something out of the norm. Be as concise as possible without padding descriptions with unnecessary adjectives or adverbs. Simple and straightforward works best and leaves time for sharing of vital information.

Even though you may be upset by the diagnosis, this is a critical time to pay close attention to everything the doctor or her associates tell you. Use *every* minute of this interaction to educate yourself. Fifteen or 30 minutes will vanish before you know it.

Written questions should also be brought along to every visit so that you feel prepared and not rushed. Prioritize what is most important to the patient's health and family's involvement in care. Subscribe to the belief that "there are no dumb questions." If you don't ask, who will? Every case is different, but don't expect your physician to guess what questions you may have.

Also be prepared to assume a reporter's role by jotting down the pertinent details of the discussion with the physician. You'll want these notes to review and report on later with family. With your doctor's permission, you might tape record the conversation, but don't rely exclusively on this means of capturing information. Always have pen and paper handy to remember highlights, even if you are given paperwork to read and write on.

Ask how to spell any unfamiliar terms in case you want to do additional research. If your doctor talks too fast for you to comprehend everything, request he slow down. Ask what he needs from you to expedite and maximize the benefits of future visits.

You can be assertive without being angry or rude. Don't hesitate to ask direct and tough questions, because at this moment, it's all about your loved one's life, and how *you* can best care for them.

"What about ..."

A sampling of questions the patient and the caregiver can build upon

63

▶ *What's the diagnosis?*

▶ *What does it mean?*

▶ *How can you be sure?*

▶ *Do we need more tests?*

▶ *Where can we get more information on the diagnosis?*

▶ *How do we go about getting a second opinion?*

▶ *What stage are we in? What does that mean?*

▶ *What is the prognosis?*

▶ *What are our medication options? Pros and cons of each?*

▶ *What about the side effects of the medication(s)?*

▶ *What can I do to minimize the side effects?*

▶ *What about alternative medicines?*

▶ *Will this be covered by insurance?*

▶ *What physical restrictions will we be facing?*

▶ *What signs, symptoms or other problems should we look for?*

▶ *What information do you have at your office on support groups for my family?*

▶ *How often do we need to come in to see you?*

▶ *Do we need a referral for another physician?*

▶ *If you were in our place, what would you do?*

Dealing with doctors

"She was not cold and clinical"

After her husband, Tom, had completed an assortment of tests, Vicky remembers going back a week later for the dreaded results: early-onset Alzheimer's.

"As soon as I looked at her, I knew. I don't remember her exact words, but she cried with us when she gave us the diagnosis. All three of us sat there and cried together. Then she left the room to let us be by ourselves. Tom just sobbed. She came back in and talked to us a little more about what to expect, though not in great detail in front of him."

Did the doctor's response help? Immensely, she says.

"She was not cold and clinical. She was very compassionate, almost like she was feeling it with us. That helped him, and it helped me because I knew I wasn't going to be alone. At that point, it was anti-climactic. 'We know what we're fighting now, and we'll fight it the best we can.' "

"They didn't tell me anything"

"When they gave us the test results, they didn't tell us anything," Peg says after her husband's initial MRI and other tests.

"I had taken him to one place, and I was less and less pleased. When one drug came out, they didn't even tell me about that. My druggist told me. I told the doctor. They had a psychologist who worked with him, and she had no tact at all. He would be so upset. I started looking for another place."

They found other care options and only then when the records were transferred did she confirm that he had early-onset Alzheimer's. By then, she had figured it out with persistent research. He saw a neurologist until he was placed in a nursing facility.

"Help me be the caregiver"

Char detailed in a journal her mother's behaviors that she had observed and took it to her mother's six-month checkups. Every time she showed it to the doctor and implored him to help.

" 'Tell me what to do. Help me be the caregiver.' "

Professionals say...

Professional caregivers assist patients and families every day on the job, yet they learn something new all the time about these conditions.

What fact about Alzheimer's, dementia or memory loss has surprised you the most? Why?

▶ How fast clients forget. Sometimes it will be things you have repeated over and over. *Latoya, 27, CNA, 2 years*

▶ Neuron studies are not that promising. *Dave, 40, executive director, 2 years*

▶ They all (no matter what stage) respond to love and a smile. *Cindy, 53, nurse, 34 years*

▶ The onset can happen at a very young age! *Marge, 50, nursing home administrator, 24 years*

▶ Its prevalence. *Ronni, R.N, 49, 28 years*

▶ How it happened to my husband. *Gloria, 54, CNA, 18 years*

▶ Everything I've ever learned about Alzheimer's and all I continue to learn surprise me because it is such an evil disease. Very cruel. *Karen, 46, developmental technician, 20 years*

▶ That a patient can have it 10 years before diagnosed. *Mary, 37, hospital social worker, 11 years*

▶ The fact that honesty is not always the best policy, that it is more acceptable not to tell the truth sometimes. *Vicki, 56, R.N., 35 years*

▶ The onset of it. My father was diagnosed at the age of 42. *Michelle, 38, 11 years*

Caregivers say...

There are moments when you wish you could read minds ... and one of those times is when a loved one is diagnosed with an illness, especially one like Alzheimer's. We can only imagine the shock within him or her, the denial, the fear, the acceptance, or depending on their stage, perhaps no real comprehension at all. Is that a curse or blessing?

How did this person react to being diagnosed, and how did he/she express or suppress their response, i.e., anger, denial, withdrawal?

- Denial
- Covered up
- No response
- Anger
- Did not understand
- Confused
- Withdrew
- Discouraged
- Willingness to seek help
- Fear for the future
- Determination
- Sadness
- Acceptance
- "Nothing I can do about it"
- Depression
- "Nothing is wrong with me"

- She knew something was wrong but didn't know anything about it at that time. *Sylvia, 58, mother, Alzheimer's, died 17 years after diagnosed*

- Grandma denied the fact, and then she wanted sympathy for the diagnosis. *Shallen, 25, grandmother, Alzheimer's*

- It was never mentioned. After being in the hospital, she couldn't live alone and needed physical therapy and more help than we could give her alone. She never argued and accepted going into a nursing home. She was actually happy with the care. *Jolene, 66, mother, dementia, died 5 years after diagnosed*

- I think she was numb. "Now what is going to happen to me?" Feeling she was alone or afraid of being alone with strangers. *Jenny, 56, mother, Alzheimer's*

- His father had it, but neither he nor his wife discussed it. *Pat, 66, husband, Alzheimer's*

- Denial. I don't think she ever accepted it. *Robert, 79, wife, Alzheimer's, died 6 years after diagnosed*

- He didn't show any emotion, seemed almost unaware it was about him. He was a quiet, gentle man. *Leora, 72, husband, Alzheimer's*

- He said we should take care of things while he can still remember. We saw a lawyer and made all of our funeral arrangements. *Edna, 83, husband, Alzheimer's, died 6 years after diagnosed*

- I don't believe Mother ever knew what was wrong. She acted giddy like an adolescent at times. My sister sort of brushed things off like getting lost driving, forgetting meetings, etc. *Norma, 81, mother, Alzheimer's, died 11 years after diagnosed; sister, Alzheimer's, died 6 years after diagnosed*

- He says he's just getting old and does not like me to tell other people he has Alzheimer's. *Maxine, 77, husband, Alzheimer's*

- Sad. He remembered his father's decline. He had been caregiver for both his parents and his wife. *Marcy, 76, father, Alzheimer's, died 5 years after diagnosed*

- At first she was concerned about the diagnosis and would repeatedly ask why she was so forgetful. As time went on, she obviously didn't remember the diagnosis, but continued to be frustrated by her poor memory. *Judith, 61, mother, Alzheimer's*

- I don't think she ever understood. She blamed any and all problems on hearing loss or me. *Anne, 67, mother, dementia, died 4 years after diagnosed*

- My dad was extremely adept before the diagnosis at hiding his symptoms. He was so far along by the time we found out that he really didn't understand or react. *Andrew, 25, father, frontal lobe dementia, diagnosed at age 51*

- She felt it was natural memory loss for her age, 81 years. *Sally, 57, mother, Alzheimer's, died 3 years after diagnosed*

"Relief that they 'weren't going crazy,' less paranoid."
Cathi, 58, mother, dementia

▶ "It won't get me, I can still do my business." He refused to alter his lifestyle and wouldn't tell anyone. *June, 66, husband, early onset Alzheimer's*

▶ No reaction. She was never told. *Nancy, 65, mother, Alzheimer's*

▶ Glad to be alive, but sad for the things he can no longer do (earn money, play golf, bowl, tennis). *Marcy, 76, husband, memory loss due to massive stroke*

▶ He needed to talk it out with many people, was very open and frank. This was in true typical form of personality for my father. *Mary, 38, father, Alzheimer's*

▶ By the time he was diagnosed, it meant nothing to him. He didn't retain information. At one point, he said, "That sounds bad." He has hardly reacted at all to having Alzheimer's. He thinks he's a "dumb boy" or "not as good as" more lately, though I know somewhere inside he knows he's not all right. He has a heavy dose of anti-depressants, and I'm sure that helps considerably. *Marlene, 68, husband, dementia/Alzheimer's*

▶ Denial, use of alcohol. *Kim, 34, grandmother, died 5 years after diagnosed*

▶ Very angry. He called the doctor names, never went back. *Sandy, 61, husband, Alzheimer's and vascular dementia*

▶ She handled it very well. She was more concerned for her boys than herself. *Kevin, 45, mother, Alzheimer's*

▶ At first he was quiet, then when he discussed it with me on the way home, it sounded as though he thought he would recover. *Norma, 81, husband, Alzheimer's*

▶ Mom was sad. She cried. She told my son and me that no matter what she said or did, she would always, always love us. *MM, 46, mother, Alzheimer's, died 5 years after diagnosed*

"She called and asked me to come and help her move into a group home." *Ann, 63, aunt, Alzheimer's, died 6 years after diagnosed*

Caregivers say...

We hear all our lives that knowledge is power, yet when we hear a diagnosis of Alzheimer's, dementia or memory loss, we often feel powerless. And in today's world, there's enough information out there that would take longer than 1,000 lifetimes to digest and comprehend, and we still wouldn't have all the answers we need ... especially *why*.

69

What did you immediately realize that you didn't know or understand about this disease?

▸ The stages

▸ Prognosis

▸ Progression

▸ What to expect

▸ Everything

▸ The cause

▸ Ups and downs

▸ How to handle it

▸ How subtle it could be

▸ How to answer his questions

▸ Every case is different

▸ How to keep her safe

▸ How much it would affect the whole family

▸ From diagnosis to death

▸ The emotions involved when a loved one is affected. *Shallen, 25, grandmother, Alzheimer's*

▸ As much as I work with families who deal with this, it was "different" for me personally. *Laurie, 47, father, dementia*

▸ The difficulty in getting simple tasks completed like baths. *John, 67, mother-in-law, Alzheimer's*

▸ That my siblings who live in other states would feel guilty that they were not able to help with Mom's regular everyday needs. *Judith, 61, mother, Alzheimer's*

"That Alzheimer's affects reasoning and logic, more than just memory." June, 66, husband, early onset Alzheimer's

▸ The doctor we started with gave her some medications. He kept giving her stronger dosages, and she became very hard to handle. We had to change doctors. *Robert, 79, wife, Alzheimer's, died 6 years after diagnosed*

▸ How hard therapy would be for him. For me, understanding the interconnection between diabetes and vascular disease throughout his body. For both of us, that recovery would be limited. *Marcy, 76, husband, memory loss due to massive stroke*

▸ How little my mother understood and how much they covered it up. How important the caregiver is and how difficult it is to change the patterns of interaction. *Ann, 49, mother, vascular dementia, died; father, Alzheimer's, died*

▸ How to accept and care for your own mother. It was hard. *Jolene, 66, mother, dementia, died 5 years after diagnosed*

▸ That I was losing my closeness with my mother. We had always enjoyed so many things together, music, sewing, cooking and shopping. *Norma, 81, mother, Alzheimer's, died 11 years after diagnosed; sister, Alzheimer's, died 6 years after diagnosed*

▸ I really knew nothing. I immediately called the Alzheimer's Association. *Ann, 63, aunt, Alzheimer's, died 6 years after diagnosed*

▸ That I wasn't invincible and needed help with her care plan. *Anne, 67, mother, dementia, died 4 years after diagnosed*

▸ How to get him off the roads and legal issues. *Marlene, 68, husband, dementia/Alzheimer's*

▸ The personal toll on the family is hard to realize until you live it. *Kim, 34, grandmother, died 5 years after diagnosed*

▸ That someone so young could be affected. *Vicky, 54, husband, early onset Alzheimer's, died 5 years after diagnosed*

▸ That it can happen to anyone, no matter how young or old. *Andrew, 25, father, frontal lobe dementia, diagnosed 2003 at age 51*

"How dependent the person becomes on others for care and safety."
Christl, 55, father, stroke and Alzheimer's

- How to help her, make her life better, keep her happy, keep her dignity. *Gayle, 59, mother, Alzheimer's, died 5 years after diagnosed*

- The amount of paranoia involved. *Jody, 47, mother, early onset Alzheimer's*

- I was not prepared for the sudden mood changes, the anger. *Catherine, 85, husband, Alzheimer's and Lewy Body*

- I wasn't sure how long we'd have or how much care she'd need. I wasn't sure the medication was available and if there was any hope. *MM, 46, mother, Alzheimer's, died 5 years after diagnosed*

- I started to find out our lives would change. *David, 69, wife, Alzheimer's*

"She could not be left alone, could no longer cook. She was the greatest cook in the world!" Sally, 57, mother, Alzheimer's, died 3 years after diagnosed

New questions I have

_____

_____

_____

_____

_____

Professionals say...

Families grapple for answers even when they may be unsure of the right questions to ask. Professional caregivers have witnessed many of the truths and misconceptions about Alzheimer's.

72

What do you want families to understand about these diseases that they may overlook or not understand?

▸ That it's nothing they did to make their loved one not remember them. *Latoya, 27, CNA, 2 years*

▸ That your loved one will change and most likely won't be who they were before. *Kalah, 48, social service assistant, four months*

▸ Live in the patients' world. Don't expect them to live in your world. *Dave, 40, executive director, 2 years*

▸ Your approach, attitude and tone are determinant of their response. *Cindy, 53, nurse, 34 years*

▸ Alzheimer's disease can only be confirmed by autopsy. There is no shame or blame. *Marge, 50, nursing home administrator, 24 years*

▸ Not all Alzheimer's patients are the same. *Sherry, 27, trainer, 2 years*

▸ Early intervention is important, that getting patients familiarized with routines of facilities and staff is important to patient's adjustment and acceptance. *Ronni, R.N, 49, 28 years*

▸ What works one day doesn't work the next, and what works with one doesn't work with another, and you're not alone. *Sharon, 55, nurse aide/driver, 15 years*

▸ An appropriate diagnosis and treatment can improve their quality of life and relationships with family. Visit your loved one. *Connie, 57, psychotherapist*

▸ That they always don't understand what is really going on with their loved one. They don't understand or know how to deal or cope with them. *Vicki, 56, R.N., 35 years*

▸ Memory impairment and how it adds to behavior. *Michelle, 48, CNA, 30 years*

▸ They don't understand that the brain connectors are severed. *Edi, social worker, 17 years*

▸ The affected cannot help it; they are not being mean or hateful. I have to wonder if deep inside, they are not in there somewhere and they are as frustrated as the rest of us. *Karen, 46, developmental technician, 20 years*

73

▸ That they may not be in the moment, not understanding, "not to sweat the small stuff." *Debi, 48, float trainer, 6 years*

▸ They are all different. *Trudy, 57, director of nursing, 30 years*

▸ Don't take anger, suspicion, paranoia or other bad behavior personally. *Susan, 58, LPN*

What misconceptions do families tend to have?

▸ That they will get better. *Pam, 44, LPN, 25 years*

▸ My family thinks my husband will get better in time, even when the doctor says it will not happen. *Gloria, 54, CNA, 18 years*

▸ The person will stay the same. *Susan, 38, R.N., 12 years*

▸ Families feel with reminders that the patient will remember. Sometimes it works, sometimes it doesn't. *Mary, 37, hospital social worker, 11 years*

▸ Thinking things will change or go back to the way they were. *Michelle, 38, 11 years*

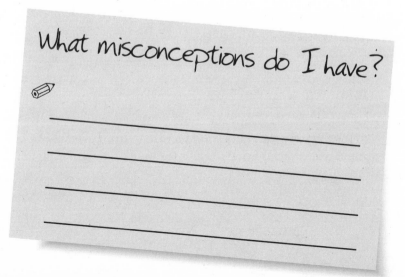

What misconceptions do I have?

The bridge from reaction to action ...

Upon hearing a diagnosis of Alzheimer's, dementia or memory loss, individuals, family and friends will react in a variety of ways at different times. Individuals may feel shock one day and anger the next or vice versa. Everyone responds differently and should understand that these unpredictable fluctuations are part of our normal human response to immediate and impending grief and loss.

We fear or dread the void that dementia and memory loss bring ... the loss of the traditions, knowledge and love that are the foundation of two-way relationships.

It's okay and *your* decision or choice to ...

▸ *Cry or shout or blame ...*

▸ *Be left alone or want to give up or feel discouraged ...*

▸ *Seek sympathy or be scared or have faith ...*

▸ *Savor favorite memories and create new ones ...*

How you react is *your* choice.

How *you* will cope with and survive this unexpected and difficult challenge will rely much on how you:

▸ *Communicate with others.*

▸ *Accept assistance when it's offered.*

▸ *Ask for assistance when you need it.*

▸ *Look for the situation's positives that are often hidden.*

▸ *Plan ahead and avoid putting off important decisions.*

▸ *Take care of yourself.*

Now's the time for you to build a bridge from immediate reaction to long-term action to protect your loved one and yourself.

The necessities
& wisdom
of planning
ahead

"He was over his head and didn't let on. I made the decision to involve an elder attorney. I found rooms full of papers he didn't know what to do with, years accumulation." Marlene, 68, husband, Alzheimer's

Caregivers say...

Gut reaction, instinct, trial and error … they're all part of the decision-making process when dealing with a family member with memory loss or dementia. Often the best advice is to plan the work and work the plan.

What was the best decision you made or thing you did in the beginning?

▸ Saw several doctors

▸ Tried experimental medication

▸ Read books

▸ Researched articles

▸ Family conference

▸ Hired part-time help

▸ Registered for Alzheimer's Association workshops

▸ Shared Alzheimer's video with family

▸ Moved parent closer

▸ Checked nursing homes

▸ Moved loved one into assisted living facility

▸ Reviewed all legal papers

▸ Updated wills

▸ Set up power-of-attorney

▸ I learned that he is actually happier and perhaps healthier living in his home of 30 years. *Christl, 55, father, stroke and Alzheimer's*

▸ Having her stay in her own home with a live-in caregiver. *Jolene, 66, mother, dementia, died 5 years after diagnosed*

▸ I talked to him about what was happening. Getting him to accept and deal with whatever happens. *Pat, 66, husband, Alzheimer's*

▸ When I saw she was having trouble with daily tasks, I kept a close eye on this and informed my brothers and sisters so they could watch out for her, too. *Jenny, 56, mother, Alzheimer's*

"Got Dad to a doctor who took the time to listen." Laurie, 47, father, dementia

▸ I had our attorney draw up financial power-of-attorney and durable power-of-attorney for health care and guardianship. *Leora, 72, husband, Alzheimer's*

▸ I hired a man to sit with him a few hours so I could get some rest. *Edna, 83, husband, Alzheimer's, died 7 years after diagnosed*

▸ I called my sister's daughter in Alaska, informing her how bad she was so she came. We packed and got rid of her condo. When we parted that day, I felt as though it was a funeral. *Norma, 81, mother, Alzheimer's, died 11 years after diagnosed; sister, Alzheimer's, died 6 years after diagnosed*

▸ I had women come in mornings so I could stop and take care of things. *Robert, 77, wife, Alzheimer's*

▸ Independent living in facility with transition to assisted living. *John, 59, mother, Alzheimer's*

▸ I went to a couple of meetings on caregiving. I tried to keep sense of humor and started the battle against it. *Robert, 79, wife, Alzheimer's, died 6 years after diagnosed*

▸ I learned not to argue or disagree with him. *Shirley, 72, husband, dementia*

▸ I continued to work, changed shifts and got a student nurse. *Anne, 67, mother, dementia, died 4 years after diagnosed*

▸ I obtained power-of-attorney so I could pay her bills and help her. *Elaine, 54, mother, Alzheimer's*

▸ I rented a large house and moved her in with my husband and myself. *Sally, 57, mother, Alzheimer's, died 3 years after diagnosed*

"Getting my brother to come to the geriatric clinic for appointments with us." Ann, 49, mother, vascular dementia, died; father, Alzheimer's, died

▸ He was willing to tell friends and relatives. This helped them relate better. *Helen, 72, husband, Alzheimer's*

▸ I didn't let her babysit my grandsons. I would take her home instead of letting her walk. *Darlene, 58, mother, Alzheimer's*

▸ I accepted the realities of the illness and try to empathize with her frustrations. *Elizabeth, 47, mother, Alzheimer's*

▸ To get her evaluated, diagnosed and consult an elder care attorney. *Kim, 34, grandmother, died 5 years after diagnosed*

▸ Not quite the beginning, but to retire, sell home and move closer to daughter. *June, 66, husband, early onset Alzheimer's*

▸ I got another job and tried to put financial things in order. *Vicky, 54, husband, early onset Alzheimer's, died 5 years after diagnosed*

▸ Sending him to adult day care twice a week. *Martha, 71, husband, cognitive decline*

▸ We realized we were going to need help in the form of a caregiver, eventually a full-care facility. *Andrew, 25, father, frontal lobe dementia, diagnosed at age 51*

▸ Making long-term plans that would benefit him. *Sandy, 61, husband, Alzheimer's and vascular dementia*

▸ I got Mom into an assisted care facility. Let her feel like it was her decision. *Kevin, 45, mother, Alzheimer's*

▸ Probably not at the beginning, but I got an Alzheimer's bracelet for him and obtained POA for health and finances. *Catherine, 85, husband, Alzheimer's and Lewy Body*

▸ I prayed for patience and strength. Never correct him or remind him of things he forgot. *Norma, 81, husband, Alzheimer's*

"I followed the advice of her friends and moved her into a group home."
Ann, 63, aunt, Alzheimer's, died 6 years after diagnosed

Let's talk about our financial, legal health

One of the harsh realities of a serious or terminal illness is that the world keeps revolving, never stopping for one event or one person. Responsibilities continue, bills must be paid, duties must be fulfilled, household chores must be juggled or delegated.

When a life-threatening event strikes a family, the immediate response is and should be to address the medical needs of the patient. However, with this crisis come new questions and worries. Time is especially crucial when dealing with Alzheimer's or memory loss because the individual may be the only one with the answers you need.

Consider the following financial and legal issues:

▸ *When was the last time we checked our medical insurance coverage? What's changed?*

▸ *What will our medical insurance cover? What's not covered?*

▸ *What must be pre-approved or pre-certified?*

▸ *Is a second opinion covered or required by the insurance?*

▸ *What's our maximum lifetime coverage? What's our co-pay?*

▸ *Does the insurance limit where we can go or what doctors we see?*

▸ *Are there limits on prescriptions? Are generics an option?*

▸ *Do we have more than one source of insurance coverage?*

▸ *Do we qualify for home health care services?*

▸ *What life insurance policies do we have? Who are the agents?*

▸ *Do we have disability insurance privately or through work? What are the requirements and limits?*

▸ *Do we have long-term care insurance privately or through work? What are the requirements and limits?*

▸ *Do we have a safety deposit box? Where is it located? Who has a key?*

▸ *Are adult children aware of where paperwork and information can be found if we need their assistance, especially if they live out of town? How will we inform them?*

▶ *Do we have a close friend or relative who can assist with some of these details?*

▶ *Do we have a valid and up-to-date will? If so, where is it and who was the attorney?*

▶ *What sources of income do we have in the event the caregiver is off work? Disability? Insurance? Investments?*

80

▶ *What's the status of all our investments? When was the last time those were evaluated? Who's the financial advisor? Do we have an accurate picture of our net worth, liabilities and assets?*

▶ *Have we set up durable power-of-attorney for all legal decisions in case we are incapacitated? If so, who is that? If not, who should it be?*

▶ *Do we have a living will and/or advanced directive that will outline our wishes in case we are incapacitated? Do we have copies we can take everywhere we go? Are our loved ones aware of our wishes?*

▶ *Have we completed funeral pre-planning? If yes, are our loved ones aware of this? What funeral home or director? Have our wishes changed since we made those arrangements? If yes, who should we contact? If we have selected cremation, are our loved ones aware of this?*

▶ *Do our loved ones understand and have they accepted our decisions on all matters related to death?*

What needs to be done?

_____
_____
_____
_____
_____
_____
_____

Caregivers say...

We're often torn between doing too much for fear of intruding into a person's life, hurting feelings or making them feel inadequate. But waiting can be emotionally and financially disastrous.

What kind of, if any, changes or plans for the future did this person begin making, positive or negative? i.e. estate planning, ignoring decisions that needed to be made.

▸ Agreed to complete power-of-attorney paperwork

▸ Made a living will

▸ Caregiver added name to bank accounts

▸ Agreed to move to senior citizen complex

▸ Agreed to estate planning

▸ Unable to make plans because of stroke damage

▸ Unable to make plans because in advanced stage

▸ Family planned together

▸ Family discussed future living arrangements

▸ Wanted to begin medications ASAP

▸ Continued with planning already in place

▸ Did nothing

▸ Nothing at first, but while she could make decisions, she told us her wishes, who she wanted to live with, etc. *Sylvia, 58, mother, Alzheimer's, died 17 years after diagnosed*

▸ Grandma decided she didn't want to be alone at all, so she stayed with my mother three and a half days and my uncle the other three and a half days a week. She also gave them power of attorney. *Shallen, 25, grandmother, Alzheimer's*

▸ I took her to visit other places to live, but she would not leave her own home. *Ellen, 69, mother*

▸ He ignored the confusion, covered it up, refused to admit it. Legal matters should have been handled prior. *Laurie, 47, father, dementia*

▸ I took over all her business as POA. I let her concentrate on just being happy. *Kevin, 45, mother, Alzheimer's*

▶ He didn't do anything, left it up to me. He did agree to sign our bodies over to the College of Medicine to help others. *Leora, 72, husband, Alzheimer's*

▶ My parents were very progressive in their planning. Having durable power-of-attorney and living wills, which we had discussed in detail, helped. *Ann, 49, mother, vascular dementia, died; father, Alzheimer's, died*

▶ He really hasn't made changes other than to stay in our house on the farm. He usually focuses on himself. His concern about me is: will I be there to take care of him and our things? *Pat, 66, husband, Alzheimer's*

▶ All decisions were made by my brother and me to ensure Dad's safety and well-being. He was not happy about not being able to drive. *Mary Ann, 62, father, Alzheimer's*

▶ Ignoring it. It was a problem. *Phil, 69, mother, dementia*

▶ He made no changes or plans. I have had to control that, but he is cooperative, i.e. funeral arrangements made and paid, lawyer discussion and power of attorney for health and property. *Maxine, 77, husband, Alzheimer's*

▶ With my and the children's insistence, we have done estate planning. Tried to get long-term care insurance for both of us. He was not accepted. I was. *Norma, 81, husband, Alzheimer's*

▶ She made arrangements for me to assume responsibilities for her financial affairs and eventually for her. *Ann, 63, aunt, Alzheimer's, died 6 years after diagnosed*

"She almost waited too late to get power of attorney, but thank God she was aware and 'with it' on the day we went to the lawyer." *MM, 46, mother, Alzheimer's, died 5 years after diagnosed*

▶ Got the wills in shape. Made a living will. Bought cemetery lots. It was something we were going to do at a younger age but didn't get to it. *Robert, 79, wife, Alzheimer's, died 6 years after diagnosed*

▶ She sold her home, gave up driving, moved here into independent living apartment, planned pre-paid funeral. It simplified things and made it easier for me to visit and assist. *John, 59, mother, Alzheimer's*

▶ He put off deciding to come live with my sister or with me. He wanted us to leave our families so he could stay in his own house. He had already taken care of estate planning. *Marcy, 76, father, Alzheimer's, died 5 years after diagnosed*

▶ None. She just withdrew. *Elizabeth, 47, mother, Alzheimer's*

▶ He is not interested in making plans, but I am making estate plans and considering future living arrangements. *Martha, 71, husband, cognitive decline*

▶ We did all the legal documents, but it was all at my urging. He didn't want people to know. He wouldn't or couldn't acknowledge that his abilities had changed. *June, 66, husband, early onset Alzheimer's*

▶ We made her sign a POA for health caregiving that assigned it to me, and not my brother who has POA over everything else. *Nancy, 65, mother, Alzheimer's*

▶ She chose to ignore it and let my mom handle everything for her. *Kim, 34, grandmother, died 5 years after diagnosed*

▶ He didn't seem as interested in our business, and we suffered. I made most of the decisions from then. *Vicky, 54, husband, early onset Alzheimer's, died 5 years after diagnosed*

▶ She knew she was dependent on me but didn't want to give up driving and her independence. *Bill, 78, wife, Alzheimer's, died 4 years after diagnosed*

▶ None. The only thing she had made was funeral arrangements for which I am grateful. *Sally, 57, mother, Alzheimer's, died 3 years after diagnosed*

▶ He refused to talk about it, so I arranged all legal papers, selling the house, buying a new house near our children and retiring early. *Sandy, 61, husband, Alzheimer's and vascular dementia*

Stop the flow of money before it's a flood of debt

The stories are becoming too familiar ... individuals with dementia or memory loss losing hundreds, if not thousands, of hard-earned dollars after a lifetime of work ... misplacing money, being targeted for scams, being overly generous with charitable giving or simply spending money uncontrollably.

Families must assume more responsibility for periodic checks on unusual spending habits of spouses, parents or grandparents, especially if they're accompanied by uncharacteristic behavior. Some people bankrupt themselves before they're diagnosed with conditions like Alzheimer's.

However, it can happen even when families think they're monitoring a loved one's spending habits after they've been diagnosed.

▸ *An individual hired a company to install an alarm system, told them he had Alzheimer's and then handed over his debit card.*

▸ *Magazine subscriptions poured in for one person with Alzheimer's because she had inadvertently agreed to a sales pitch over the phone, and it took the family months to stop the flood of bills.*

▸ *One woman's church stopped by weekly only to pick up donation checks though church members never inquired about her health or offered to give her a ride to services.*

We can hope that those businesses and organizations that truly care for our loved ones, and have had a long relationship with them, will notice unusual spending behavior. However, we cannot rely on that in a world that, thanks to technology, bombards us with more offers to buy and contribute than ever before.

Consider taking these immediate steps for a loved one with dementia or memory loss with these consumer protection options direct from the United States Federal Trade Commission (*www.ftc.gov*):

▸ *Register phone numbers at www.donotcall.gov or 1-888-382-1222 from the phone you want to register. You will receive fewer telemarketing calls within three months of registering your number. It will stay in the registry for five years or until it is disconnected or you take it off the registry. After five years, you will be able to renew your registration.*

▸ *Register names and addresses with the Direct Marketing Association* to opt out of mailings at Mail Preference Service, P.O. Box 643, Carmel, NY 10512 or online at www.the-dma.org/consumers/offmailinglist.html. *When you register with this service, your name will be put on a "delete" file and made available to direct-mail marketers. However, your registration will not stop mailings from organizations that are not registered with the Mail Preference Service.*

▶ *The credit bureaus offer a toll-free number that enables you to "opt-out" of having pre-approved credit offers sent to you for two years. Call 1-888-5-OPTOUT (567-8688) or visit www.optoutprescreen.com for more information. When you call, you'll be asked for personal information, including your home telephone number, your name, and your Social Security number. The information you provide is confidential and will be used only to process your request to opt out of receiving pre-screened offers of credit.*

▶ *In addition, you can notify the three major credit bureaus that you do not want personal information about you shared for promotional purposes — an important step toward eliminating unsolicited mail. Write a letter asking them to limit the amount of information the credit bureaus will share about you. Send your letter to each of the three major credit bureaus:*

  ▶ *Equifax, Inc., Options, P.O. Box 740123, Atlanta, GA 30374-0123*

  ▶ *Experian, Consumer Opt-Out, 701 Experian Parkway, Allen, TX 75013*

  ▶ *TransUnion, Name Removal Option, P.O. Box 505, Woodlyn, PA 19094*

Evaluate these other financial commitments in meeting your specific situation, and hopefully in cooperation with the individual with dementia or memory loss, to avoid financial ruin:

▶ *Set up health care power of attorney and durable power of attorney.*

▶ *Cancel most or all credit cards.*

▶ *Contact financial advisors.*

▶ *Set up automatic payments and deposits.*

▶ *Account for all checks written.*

▶ *Create joint accounts. The good news: adding someone to the individual's checking account provides for closer scrutiny of checks written and other withdrawals of funds. The bad news: this second person could become liable for debts incurred by the individual with dementia or memory loss.*

Caregivers say...

When we sincerely try to do the "right thing" for loved ones, they may not always understand. With conditions such as memory loss or dementia, it can be frustrating because impaired and decreased cognitive functions can make them defensive, suspicious or uncooperative; push them further into denial, or accelerate their lack of any response or apathy.

86

How did planning or lack of it affect the situation?

▸ Extremely helpful

▸ Guaranteed his safety

▸ Making funeral plans helped

▸ Saved the cost of her funeral later

▸ Caregiver took over his finances to care for him

▸ Had no reaction

▸ Should have made her stop driving earlier

▸ Helped ease caregiver's worries

▸ Putting a plan into place helped everyone

▸ Settled her affairs without concerning her

▸ Should have gotten power-of-attorney paperwork completed earlier

▸ Spouse had to make all decisions by herself

▸ She was grateful someone else was taking care of everything

▸ It all worked out

▸ Sometimes it would become annoying, because it was always the same questions, and she would not recognize it at times. *Shallen, 25, grandmother, Alzheimer's*

▸ It was hard to figure out what to do. There's lots of work to do living on a farm, and I don't know if I can do it all. *Pat, 66, husband, Alzheimer's*

▸ It helped because he was not able to make decisions. *Leora, 72, husband, Alzheimer's*

▸ I control her life totally. *David, 69, wife, Alzheimer's*

"It gives me more peace of mind." Martha, 71, husband, cognitive decline

▶ We shifted the load to others, and we all gladly adapted to help Mom. *Cathi, 58, mother, dementia*

▶ The delay allowed him to have more car mishaps. He got lost driving home. He lost too much weight by not eating. He must have been lonely. *Marcy, 76, father, Alzheimer's, died 5 years after diagnosed*

▶ We were very fortunate that Mom virtually agreed with our decisions to make changes. *Judith, 61, mother, Alzheimer's*

▶ I felt totally responsible for her, but it is working out. *Elaine, 54, mother, Alzheimer's*

▶ It hindered in that he didn't realize at first that he really wasn't capable. *Helen, 72, husband, Alzheimer's*

▶ I had to hide that I was doing tax preparation and other bill paying. *Marlene, 68, husband, dementia/Alzheimer's*

▶ It meant she did not resist our help, but it made me miss her more. *Elizabeth, 47, mother, Alzheimer's*

▶ Actually, it was probably easier that way. She was very trusting and docile. *Kim, 34, grandmother, died 5 years after diagnosed*

▶ It was a load of responsibility for me. Two sons lived far away and the one nearby still needed help himself. *Marcy, 76, husband, memory loss due to massive stroke*

▶ It helped greatly. My brother is a lawyer, and Dad was very intent on having things well planned. That was part of his personality always. *Mary, 38, father, Alzheimer's*

▶ It was the best decision for him but not what I saw as my future. There was so much more I wanted to do. *Sandy, 61, husband, Alzheimer's and vascular dementia*

"I don't think it did much for her, but it did help me near her death." Robert, 79, wife, Alzheimer's, died 5 years after diagnosed

Will you sign on for the proactive or procrastinator plan?

Power of attorney, estate planning, guardianship, long-term care and HIPAA are generally not the main course of conversation at the Thanksgiving dinner table. However, if that's the only time you can get the family together to discuss these important issues that are crucial to caring for a loved one with dementia or memory loss, then maybe save it for after dessert.

A local attorney frequently speaks to dozens of families at workshops sponsored by the Alzheimer's Association. Families of individuals with dementia or memory loss must face basic legal and financial necessities. These are packed with complex layers of legalities that represent laws intended to protect individuals.

There are many misconceptions about an array of terminology that peppers legal conversation about Alzheimer's. Many adult children have no idea what to do for their parents, especially if they live out of town. If no provisions have been put in place, families must often work their way through a maze of rules to address the assets, privacy, rights and health of their loved one. To add to the confusion, every state adopts different formulas.

There are two approaches to advance directives: proactive tools or the procrastinator package.

The best advice?

▶ *Don't wait for a crisis to make important financial and legal decisions.*

▶ *Deal with private matters before they become public.*

▶ *Avoid a race to see which relative "gets there first" to claim money or guardianship.*

▶ *Don't assume the oldest or Mom and Dad's favorite child is the best to oversee these matters. Pick the best person for the job.*

In other words, avoid the procrastinator route because it costs more money, time and hardship, and often goes against what the individual with dementia or memory loss would have wanted.

The proactive tools include the creation of living wills, health care power of attorney, and property power of attorney and trusts, either revocable or irrevocable.

Living wills provide the legal vehicle in which the individual can determine if they want to be maintained on life support or if heroic medical measures are used in saving their life. This will ease the family's responsibility in being forced to make those end-of-life decisions under difficult emotional circumstances.

89

The health care power of attorney gives the assigned caregiver the authority to be informed about the patient's medical history, preferred providers and pharmacist, and insurance information in making the best decisions on behalf of the patient.

The property or durable power of attorney gives the assignee the power to act on behalf of the individual with dementia or memory loss on matters of personal property, including all financial concerns.

While one individual, such as an adult child, may be assigned both powers, many families find that choosing two people, one for each responsibility, works best in keeping "checks and balances" and eases the burden on each.

A revocable or irrevocable trust can outline the individual's wishes on living arrangements, such as being moved to a nursing home or other setting. Patients' rights are protected under the federal Nursing Home Reform Act.

Pre-planned funeral arrangements — whether pre-paid or not — can also save families considerable stress and money. This way, the wishes of the individual can be honored, such as burial location or the decision to be cremated.

People often don't want to take the time or incur the expense of planning ahead, but to do so is a fraction of the cost of being swept up in the legal system when emotions are high.

The whole reason of planning ahead is to avoid disputes.

What is HIPAA all about?

HIPAA is one of the most widely used and least understood acronyms in our modern society. You've likely signed off on this legislation every time you see any of your medical providers. You're not alone if you don't have a clue what it really means.

This federal law affects virtually every medical interaction in this country. Understanding this law is especially important for caregivers because your ability to make informed decisions on behalf of your loved one relies on obtaining the information you need about treatments, etc.

According to the United States Department of Health and Human Services (HHS), *"To improve the efficiency and effectiveness of the health care system, the Health Insurance Portability and Account-ability Act (HIPAA) of 1996, Public Law 104-191, included 'Administrative Simplification' provisions that required HHS to adopt national standards for electronic health care transactions. At the same time, Congress recognized that advances in electronic technology could erode the privacy of health information."*

And what does this mean?

Basically, it protects the privacy of your health care records.

Here are a couple of related topics addressed by the HHS:

Question: If someone has health care power of attorney for an individual, can they obtain access to that individual's medical record?

Answer: Yes, an individual that has been given a health care power of attorney will have the right to access the medical records of the individual related to such representation to the extent permitted by the HIPAA Privacy Rule at 45 CFR 164.524. However, when a physician or other covered entity reasonably believes that an individual, including an unemancipated minor, has been or may be subjected to domestic violence, abuse or neglect by the personal representative, or that treating a person as an individual's personal representative could endanger the individual, the covered entity may choose not to treat that person as the individual's personal representative, if in the exercise of professional judgment, doing so would not be in the best interests of the individual.

Question: Does the HIPAA Privacy Rule change the way in which a person can grant another person health care power of attorney?

Answer: No. Nothing in the Privacy Rule changes the way in which an individual grants another person power of attorney for health care decisions. State law (or other law) regarding health care powers of attorney continue to apply. *The intent of the provisions regarding personal representatives was to complement, not interfere with or change, current practice regarding health care powers of attorney or the designation of other personal representatives. Such designations are formal, legal actions which give others the ability to exercise the rights of, or make treatment decisions related to, an individual. The Privacy Rule provisions regarding personal representatives generally grant persons, who have authority to make health care decisions for an individual under other law, the ability to exercise the rights of that individual with respect to health information.*

In other words, check with your attorney, insurance or health-care provider to decipher any and all legalese that affects you.

Paperwork to complete

_____

_____

_____

_____

_____

_____

_____

_____

_____

_____

Paper piles...

"Plan it out"

"It was hard in the beginning," Sue recalls. "I would sneak it into the conversation. 'Gee, Mom, if this should ever happen, what would you like?' I was able to get her to give me medical power of attorney and for property as well. She didn't fight me on that. I was very fortunate as opposed to many people I know who go through experiences like that."

She advises families to read everything they can get their hands on and start planning. Now that dementia and memory loss can be diagnosed much earlier, the individual's involvement in planning their own future is a huge advantage.

"I wish we had had that opportunity to have her more involved. We didn't realize ..." She encourages families to take advantage of training and educational opportunities, such as those offered by the Alzheimer's Association and other groups. "Being in a crisis is not the best time to be making those decisions. Plan it out and know where you're headed. The resources are out there."

She's also found her role as a healthcare professional to be a tremendous boon.

"I really think that helped me. I have contacts. I know where the resources are. I know when things don't seem right." Laughing, she recalls the many headaches Medicaid paperwork has generated. "Even that is a challenge for me. I have probably more insight than the average person. I certainly have an appreciation for the complexities of the healthcare system and how it is so fragmented."

There's often no insurance coverage for assisted living and private care, which can be less expensive than nursing home services. Families often face huge out-of-pocket expenses for those services.

"Unfortunately, assisted living is very expensive, but luckily we have the means to do that. A lot of people can't do that. They have no options. How do we get more funding for people to get assistance and have the resources to get some in-home help and respite care? Certainly, volunteers can visit and let the caregiver go to the store. I was always able to arrange it so that I could work." She credits her sister and sister-in-law for assisting in her mother's care on a regular basis for a couple of years.

"You have to have that kind of help to do this. Many people don't have those resources. Long-term care planning is important. People don't imagine they'll ever need it."

93

"I learned the hard way"

When Peg talks with other families dealing with dementia and memory loss, she tells it like it is after coping with her husband's early-onset Alzheimer's.

"There are things I did wrong. I didn't do the legal stuff right. I learned the hard way."

Her husband had wanted to make sure she had no problems. They had seen an attorney to put the house in her name. That lawyer was okay for that step, but she needed someone who specialized in elder law. She found out a little too late about getting the proper diagnosis, the expense of nursing homes and how to properly register her husband for Medicaid.

"I'm gung ho about getting to a lawyer and getting the proper things done. You can really be in trouble."

"You have to look ahead"

"You cope with what you need to do now," says Char, after dealing with her mother-in-law's and mother's Alzheimer's. "At the same time, you have to look ahead in terms of what could be a plan."

She and her husband, Jim, visited different care facilities to plan for the future. Get your name on the list immediately so that you have options, she advises.

Jim says it's easy for families to run through all their financial resources very quickly if they've not planned ahead. It will be helpful if you try to involve the individual with dementia or memory loss. This is most effective in the early stages when that person can contribute financial information to the planning process.

"It creates a huge emotional toll if it's not taken care of."

"We need to prepare for our own longevity"

94

Pam watched her parents' hard-earned life savings and personal belongings evaporate to pay for her mother's nursing home care. The anger and sadness she felt in coping with her mother's dementia multiplied, and though there was nothing she could do for her mother, this long moment in time planted a seed deep within Pam to make sure other families didn't suffer the same anguish.

The four siblings noticed their mother was somewhat forgetful during phone conversations, but they attributed it to the fact that she was 80 years old. Then one day, she ended up 20 miles from home with no idea where or why she was there, though she used the excuse that she was going to the store and got distracted.

The adult children pooled their resources to move her into a senior facility for a couple of years until she needed more supervision and was admitted to a nursing home. Pam called regularly, but her mom wouldn't talk about the present, only telling stories that happened 40 or 50 years earlier.

"I guess I chose to feel good about those conversations and to laugh as opposed to being upset that she was living in the past. Sometimes during those conversations, I would ask what she had for lunch, and she didn't remember lunch had occurred."

The reality of dementia hit the day when Pam and her brother visited. Their mother recognized him but kept looking at Pam and saying, "You look like a daughter of mine." This happened numerous times in a half hour. That was eight years into the dementia and three years before she died.

As she continued her decline, the mother dismissed Pam and others because she didn't recognize them and didn't want anybody around her. She slept a lot. The last time Pam visited, a couple of years before her death, "She didn't have a clue who I was, and I was an agitation to her. She would tell me, 'You can go away now.' Those were the last face-to-face meetings I had with her."

How did that affect her?

"The day she recognized my brother and not me, that was devastating. How could she not recognize me? I was the baby of the family. There was a lot of guilt associated with this whole thing, guilt that she was 200 miles away. Originally, she wanted so badly to live with us. I told her, 'Mom, that's not realistic in our ability to care for you.' "

Like millions of other adults, Pam found herself in the "sandwich generation," caught between the needs of her parent and her own busy teen-aged children.

"I felt guilty that Mom wanted to live with us, and without sacrificing a ton for my own family, I didn't see that as being possible. There's a lot of guilt associated with that." The money necessary to have someone care for her mother in their home was prohibitive as she and her husband prepared to send their children to college. Her mother didn't want to live in a nursing home in Pam's community. That left few options.

In the beginning, Pam felt guilt, yet accepted the disease. "Why my mom? Why not my mom?" It was an attitude. The last few years were also guilt-ridden because she didn't visit.

"She was more comfortable without me there. I didn't see the point of driving three and a half hours to talk to a nurse to see how she was doing when I could do that over the phone. That's what I did, but I felt guilty not going to see her."

She was torn emotionally about her loyalty to her mother and to her family. To whom should she devote her time, energy and money? In retrospect, she believes she made the right decision. However, from all these lessons emerged the desire to make sure other families didn't share her experience.

"People shouldn't have to deal with the emotional and financial issues of 'What's right?' and 'Where's my loyalty?' Our parents and *we* need to prepare for our own longevity." Society has advanced so much medically that a heart attack or stroke won't easily kill us, and certainly Alzheimer's won't. "We're living longer and dying slower. We need to prepare for that fact. The greatest gift a person can give their children is preparing for their own old age."

Pam retired from retail and wanted to create a new career for herself. She had worked since she 10 years old, starting in the family restaurant. Her parents had worked more than 40 years to save for retirement, and it was depleted almost immediately after her mother went into the nursing home.

She remembers her mother's estate sale and so many special objects being sold. "That was a hurtful day," she says, her eyes filling with tears.

The value of her mother's estate upon her death? $218 ... the interest from her pre-paid funeral arrangements.

After learning much from her own experience, Pam opted to enter the insurance field and focus on long-term care policies.

Most families can't begin to comprehend the financial toll of Alzheimer's and related diseases if they've never experienced it. Men and women are different, she has found. She believes that men are more in denial, based on what they've told her. She's had many men tell her they're *never* going to a nursing home. She responds that long-term care insurance may be the only thing that keeps them out of a nursing home. What would happen if they had dementia, even if they're in perfect health otherwise?

" 'That won't happen to *me.*' I've had two men tell me in the last month that they have a gun and they'll commit suicide before they'll accept Alzheimer's. I told them, 'You may have a gun, but if you have dementia, you may not know what to do with it.' "

Women are generally more concerned and interested because they'll likely assume more of the caregiver role for a parent or spouse. Women are also more willing to discuss options for the day *they* need assistance. Some people are very quick to say they don't want their children participating in their care.

"A couple of months in a nursing home can wipe a family out financially," Pam says. "As a society, we're not prepared with 78 million baby boomers. This country and economy have never seen anything like what will happen. Nobody's prepared, not even the government. Medicaid cannot be relied on to provide coverage for the boomers. People have to take responsibility for their own longevity and healthcare because 'here we come!' "

Medicare won't save the day, and 65 is not the magic retirement number anymore. People can't rely on company or retirement health coverage, she explains. Families need to understand what long-term planning really means. The definition has changed. Individual and group health insurance is for acute care, not long-term care. Medicare pays for skilled care in a nursing home setting, and it will only pay so much for so long.

These are the harsh realities that she shares as a child of a parent requiring long-term care services. This future demand also means many employees will miss work to care for family members, which will dramatically affect this nation's productivity. Individuals need to protect the assets they've accumulated throughout a lifetime of working.

"The longer we live, the more we wear out."

Most senior care is offered outside of the nursing home setting, i.e., assisted living facilities, the home or adult day care. Long-term care policies offer the freedom to choose the kind of care we want. Individuals can only get Medicaid benefits by spending down assets to poverty levels.

"You have to be impoverished and the government sends you to a nursing home. There are no choices. There are fewer Medicaid beds available now than ever before. That closest bed may be a hundred miles away."

Families can be torn apart by lack of planning. Inheritances vanish. People generally want to leave gifts to their children, favorite charities and church, but there will be nothing left of their estate if they don't plan. Guilt and accusations can erupt as many decisions are made in a crisis situation. One of Pam's siblings didn't agree with the others about their mother's care and is estranged.

"Planning eases the burden on loved ones. It's not actually preparing for death but really for life. Plan to live the way you want to live. You'll pay one way or another, and later will always cost more," she adds.

What did they do with the $218 their mother left behind?

Three of the four siblings and their spouses went out for a memorable evening, told stories and remembered the good times. It was by no means disrespectful. Pam smiles.

"And if Mom had been there, she would have been the life of the party."

97

One family's on-the-job lessons to cope with Alzheimer's behavior

"When you're raising children, they continue to learn. With Alzheimer patients, they forget. They don't connect things," says Jim. "My mother used to tell me, *'It's you guys who have the problem, not me.'* You can't rationalize with them."

Jim and Char share some of the techniques they've learned in caring for two parents with Alzheimer's disease:

▸ *They can't separate junk from important mail. Have all mail forwarded to the caregiver.*

▸ *Check the least likely places for missing items. They found bills and her mother's purse under a mattress and a ring in an aspirin bottle. "They go to great lengths to hide things and then forget."*

▸ *Put a small amount of money in an envelop in a purse or wallet so the individual has some cash. She would buy a bunch of bananas and then write the check for $50 or $75 to get the rest back in cash.*

▸ *Take away all credit cards and checkbooks. They found her check registry, and nothing was written or ever balanced. She went through thousands of dollars with no idea why or how she used the checks.*

▸ *Have the name of the individual with dementia or memory loss taken off the mailing lists of all organizations seeking donations. There are some that will take advantage of one donation and barrage the donor with requests.*

▸ *Arrange for automatic payments and deposits.*

▸ *If they're still living on their own, make sure they're eating properly by preparing a week's worth of meals ahead of time. Contact services like Meals on Wheels to assist.*

▸ *Make day-to-day adaptations to survive, and sift out real issues that need to be dealt with immediately.*

▸ *You have to tell lies at times to keep them calm. Keep things and answers simple. Changing the subject quickly will divert them.*

▸ *"Life is short. Value each day, especially in Alzheimer's. Try to find humor. You have to have some laughing time."*

Coping:
It's full of trials
and errors and
successes

"He's in denial and depressed. He's forgotten how to do things he always did. He still thinks he'll wake up feeling 'right' again."
Pat, 66, husband, Alzheimer's

Just talking...

(Caregiver and client responses and reactions are in italics.)
At the sixth and final session, the Alzheimer's Association facilitators ask the pairs of participants how they've benefited from
this educational and support group experience.

"I enjoy everybody," announces one client.

*"I do appreciate being here," says another. "I get something every
single time. The little ideas take a load off my shoulders, the things I
beat myself up over. This gives me a break."*

"I like it because it makes everybody happy," a client says.

*A sister says her family keeps everyone going as they help their
brother deal with his Alzheimer's. "If he makes fun of himself, we all
jump in. And he forgets anyway ..."*

The caregivers gather with Bonnie again ...

*"My husband said we can't miss this meeting." The wife said his
brother refuses to believe he has Alzheimer's.*

*One husband couldn't remember how to open the cell phone and
what to press once he reached the keypad.*

A spouse tried making a phone call on a television remote control.

*One had to tell a neighbor to go over and put the person's phone
back on the hook. One family member bought him the fanciest phone,
and he can't use it because it's too complex.*

Bonnie asks what each of them will take from this group
experience.

*One says she's learned that there's only so much they can carry as
caregiver, and that it's a learning process for all of them. "In the beginning, I was extremely frustrated, but I've learned a lot. You all gave me
such feelings. There's help. I'm not alone. People not associated with
this don't understand."*

A wife announces that her husband's been moving dishes around.

*That triggers an avalanche of similar experiences: one throws away
silverware, another is constantly moving things, another is digging out
old shirts to wear, and yet another is putting dirty dishes in the cabinet.*

Bonnie nods.

"Things are not registering the way they should be. The brain is broken. If you have real valuable stuff, put it in a safe deposit box. It will happen. We don't know why they behave in this way."

The longest memories are still alive, she explains. They go back in time believing that's where they are. They don't see themselves and won't recognize their reflections, so that's why caregivers are encouraged to cover mirrors. They get to the point where they don't recognize that "old woman or old man" living with them as their spouse.

Is Alzheimer's the actual cause of death?

Alzheimer's makes the body forget to eat or breathe eventually, she explains. Many become totally bedridden, and those families face the decision of feeding tubes. For years, it was said people didn't die of Alzheimer's. Now it's reported they do. People are living longer with or without Alzheimer's.

Thanks to this group, one spouse says it's been easier to cope knowing she's not alone in what she's experiencing.

"I remember Bonnie saying not to press him," says another, as she learned to stop repeating herself. "Don't you think our group gave us the courage to try?" A chorus of voices agree, thankful for the many tips they've learned along the way.

Another wife tells of how she and her husband went to church and came home. She fixed coffee while he got the paper and dozed off. When he woke up, he said it was time for church and was adamant about it.

"If I had a sense of losing myself," Bonnie says, "what would I do? I'd at first be angry. Ordering is a way to control everything. We can't just ask them what they're thinking. Their behaviors make sense to them, and if they create their own order, then that helps them. It's all about being good enough. Abstract thinking doesn't make sense, and they may be happy just watching TV."

"While they're watching, we can put things away."

Yes, a sense of humor comes to the rescue again.

This group has meshed so well that they gather with Jenn and Bonnie once before the end of the year and again in January. The first one was a perfect opportunity to plan how the families will face the holidays.

"I wish I knew how old my kids are," says one client.

Another one looks forward to all the noise of grandkids because the house is so quiet all the time.

When asked how many grandchildren he had, a client pauses, his lips counting. He settles for "a lot."

Bonnie reminds caregivers to observe how their loved ones function in different social settings. Some may still be "social butterflies" even if they can't remember names. Others will need a quiet place as a refuge in large groups, even if it's just family.

Planning for the holidays is stressful for everyone. She advises everyone to make it easy on themselves this year.

That may be the best gift for everyone.

In January, the caregivers converse with Bonnie ... *A wife says it's been hard to see her husband go through his dementia after he saw his own parents live long lives with all their faculties until the end.*

Another laments how her husband had always been so positive and now sees everything with a negative attitude and paranoia. It's finally registered with him that he's going to die, and "he's not interested in prolonging his life because 'I'll be more stupid at the end.' "

Bonnie explains that personality changes are the hardest to adjust to in a relationship. Grief can begin even before a diagnosis, not necessarily wallowing in it, but acknowledging it.

Another says her father has become "fun again" after taking a new medication. That's eased everybody's stress.

Depression often goes with Alzheimer's, Bonnie says. Medication can ease the depression and increase the overall ability to function. However, it may help with one aspect but create other problems. Caregivers must be vigilant in checking with their physicians and pharmacists on dosages and side effects.

"The doctors are not living with our people, and they don't understand our everyday life."

"Nobody knows your people as well as you do," she says. "The caregivers know better the everyday realities and what their loved ones are capable of doing for as long as possible."

Caregivers will encounter ongoing grief as the relationship continues to dissolve under the effect of dementia and memory loss. While they're trying to get through 24 hours, they often don't realize what is vanishing every day.

Enjoy and hold onto the glimpses of the way they used to be, but don't focus too much on past capabilities.

"This is a courageous group of people. We've got a number to call."

Acceptance isn't easy

Dementia or memory loss have to be acknowledged for the unique challenges and opportunities they offer.

That's the top lesson Alisha learned while working with the elderly population before she accepted the job of patient and family services coordinator at a chapter of the Alzheimer's Association. From feeding and bathing to planning activities at assisted living facilities, she seized every opportunity to learn about this unique age group, especially those individuals coping with dementia or memory loss.

She tells families, in non-scientific terms, that it's a physical disease, that protein gums up brain cells, and it's something this person couldn't help. Many times, she's witnessed those light-bulb moments when family members realize, "Oh, it's physical."

However, everyone has to come to terms with the diagnosis in their own way. Nobody can force someone to accept this news. It can take years to grasp the emotions involved because it's a disease of long duration. She advises that to be angry or in denial for years is not healthy. That's when she suggests they attend support groups and/or see a qualified mental health counselor or therapist. It's important to talk through the emotions because, sure enough, someone else is going through the same experience.

"We know what you're going through because we've seen many families, not that yours isn't special. Be supportive of whatever stage your loved one is in. Realize 'This is how I can help now.' "

There exists no magic wand to say "accept this." Alisha acknowledges that even with all her experience and education, she wouldn't be ready to accept this news about her own loved one, and "I teach this." There's a great deal to accept along the way, not just the disease itself.

"There are many things we need to do to keep our person safe. It's all draining. What do we need to do for a family?" It's important not to get wrapped up in the disabilities but in the individual's abilities, what they *can* do.

"If you keep looking at the negatives, you're going to get bogged down in the rest of *their* life. If you can look at it and say, 'Hey, they still can do that,' let's embrace it now. You may not have that next month."

Caregivers say...

It takes time to absorb shocking, shattering news about someone you love. For some, it soaks in the same day, others, days, weeks, months later. New realities then hit us, almost forcing us to put our deep emotions aside for the moment ... which can be good or bad.

How did you adjust or accept this news/diagnosis over time? What concerns did you have?

- Life expectancy
- Diet
- Medication
- Leaving her alone
- How to adapt to her changes
- Maintaining an "I can do it" attitude
- Worried about money
- Didn't want a nursing home
- Getting her to move
- How to find proper care
- How to prevent him from driving
- Slow adjustment for everyone
- Continuous adjustment
- Accepted it head-on
- Education
- Keeping a close eye on her

- Getting involved
- Safety
- Taking over day-to-day responsibilities
- Knowing I couldn't care for her at home
- Her suspicions and paranoia
- She could not tell me if she was hurting
- She didn't understand what was happening to her
- Extended independent living as long as possible
- Extended assisted living as long as possible
- How long would it be before she got really bad?
- Will we still be able to enjoy life?
- Her happiness

▸ Accepted it calmly because now we knew what we were dealing with. *Laurie, 47, father, dementia*

▸ Have gone to several doctors, had MRIs. It's been a process of eliminating any other causes. I am concerned that I can handle taking care of him. *Pat, 66, husband, Alzheimer's*

▸ I just went day by day and hoped I would do what was best for both of us. I was concerned financially and wondered when and where he would go eventually. *Leora, 72, husband, Alzheimer's*

▸ I accepted it for what it was. Stressful to watch someone you love diminish mentally. Concerns about adequate care, driving. *Mary Ann, 62, father, Alzheimer's*

▸ It was hard to get other family members to understand or to help out. *Nettie, 51, father, Alzheimer's*

▸ With Mother, I feared for her safety. She lived alone after Daddy died. Her home was 20 miles away. I had two teenagers and lived on a farm. With my sister, I felt lost and I needed to take care for her, but being 100 miles away I relied on her ex-husband and phone calls. Her daughter took her to Alaska to care for her for about two years. We visited her several times and as she progressed, I advised my niece to put her in an Alzheimer's unit at a nursing home. *Norma, 81, mother, Alzheimer's, died 11 years after diagnosed; sister, Alzheimer's, died 6 years after diagnosed*

▸ I had to accept work, no choice keeping our bills paid. (I didn't realize) how important I was in the whole thing. *Roseann, 72, husband, dementia, died 10 years after diagnosed*

"It is a continual, daily and more frequent adjustment. You don't give enough space (on the survey form) to list concerns." Ann, 49, mother, vascular dementia, died; father, Alzheimer's, died

▸ I didn't want to accept it but didn't have time to think of me. I knew the job was going to be hard. I had heart surgery. Our children watched her while I was in the hospital. *Robert, 79, wife, Alzheimer's, died 6 years after diagnosed*

▸ To help her find joy when and where she could, to let her know she was loved. *Ann, 63, aunt, Alzheimer's, died 6 years after diagnosed*

▸ One day at a time. How do I cope? I am 10 years older than her, and she is in good health. I never stop worrying. *David, 69, wife, Alzheimer's*

▸ We anticipated the news. I was concerned about how caring for Dad would affect our family life. *Marcy, 76, father, Alzheimer's, died 5 years after diagnosed*

▸ I am the oldest (daughter) of five and it seemed natural that I would be her caregiver. My children are grown. My husband was retired and could help with taking Mom to appointments, etc. *Judith, 61, mother, Alzheimer's*

▸ I stood back and watched how it affected her, and I went to the Alzheimer's Association and talked to them. *Elaine, 54, mother, Alzheimer's*

▸ The finality of the illness has taken the longest to accept. I still grieve as she slips from one level down to the next. I still miss her. *Elizabeth, 47, mother, Alzheimer's*

▸ Moment by moment. Grief is like an onion: you peel off (work through) one layer, think you're done and then come to realize there is yet another layer after layer. Concern for mother, the caregiver. *Mary, 38, father, Alzheimer's*

▸ We were just concerned about how and where to care for her and having the financial means to take care of her. *Kim, 34, grandmother, died 5 years after diagnosed*

▸ I was caught up in her dependence on me and had to adjust. *Bill, 78, wife, Alzheimer's, died 4 years after diagnosed*

"Plan events later in the day. Dad's arguing with Mom when he knows he can't!" Cathi, 58, mother, dementia

▶ It's a continued re-adjustment. Concerns were financial, how to live life. Will we still be able to enjoy life? *June, 66, husband, early onset Alzheimer's*

▶ How to avoid it myself. *Nancy, 65, mother, Alzheimer's*

▶ I adjusted/accepted by doing lots of research. A major concern was what we would do with our business and if I would find another job. *Vicky, 54, husband, early onset Alzheimer's, died 5 years after diagnosed*

▶ The greatest challenge is determining when the time would be to place her in a long-term care facility. *Brian, 47, mother, Alzheimer's*

▶ There really wasn't much of an adjustment because we had already been living it. We now had a name to associate it with. My concerns were primarily with my mom and my brother. *Andrew, 25, father, frontal lobe dementia, diagnosed at age 51*

▶ Some resentment that he had not taken care of himself earlier in life and that *my* retirement would never happen. *Marcy, 76, husband, memory loss due to massive stroke*

▶ My main concern was about myself. I have multiple sclerosis. Who was going to help me now? *Martha, 71, husband, cognitive decline*

▶ How to manage. I was angry and still am that my life would be given up to this terrible disease. *Sandy, 61, husband, Alzheimer's and vascular dementia*

▶ Took everything in stride. Made a plan and attacked it, plan for financial, medical and ways to maximize the quality of her life. Got as much information and support as possible. *Kevin, 45, mother, Alzheimer's*

▶ I gradually assumed all responsibility. It wasn't too hard because I had always done about 80 percent of the management and work. *Catherine, 85, husband, Alzheimer's and Lewy Body*

▶ I didn't want to believe it. I knew I couldn't put her in a nursing home when it came to that. I wasn't sure what my role would be. *MM, 46, mother, Alzheimer's, died 5 years after diagnosed*

▶ I didn't tell anyone except our son and daughter. Outsiders didn't catch on for the first year. Even then and now, lots of acquaintances don't notice. *Norma, 81, husband, Alzheimer's*

"I get frustrated and he gets mad at me"

Ed and Shirley looked forward to celebrating their 50th wedding anniversary. Unfortunately, Ed will have to rely on Shirley to be his memory when the event's over.

Despite Ed's stroke-related dementia, they've fared well as a couple, especially since Shirley didn't like him when they met while bowling. Fortunately, she changed her mind. They married and had four kids. He became a research chemist, and she worked in retail and restaurants through the years.

A few years ago, a stroke affected Ed's speech, and it wasn't until sometime later that they realized something was wrong with his short-term memory. Shirley says she wishes they would have detected it sooner.

Ed asks her if it would have made any difference. She says probably not, but he could have started medication sooner. However, she admits his long-term memory is better than hers.

"I can't remember that far back. I think we moved too many times to remember."

That probably keeps them balanced.

Ed's overall health issues have kept them from traveling as much as they had hoped at this stage of their lives together. Their children's families are very supportive and fill in when she needs to get out of the house for a while.

"I get so sick and tired of sitting for doctor appointments. We have seven doctors we go to. I come home more physically exhausted from sitting in doctor's offices than I do from working six hours a day." She's a bit of a compulsive knitter who always has yarn and needles at hand, which helps her arthritis and keeps her from going crazy during the waits. "It calms me down."

She says he forgets to shower, and she has to sneak dirty clothes out when she can convince him to clean up. Ed says he does all right especially since he stays home most of the time.

"I always comb my hair. I used to shave every day, but now only when it moves me. I brush my teeth once a day, not twice. When I worked, I showered every day. But now that I'm not working, maybe twice a week."

He doesn't think he has much trouble sleeping. She says he sleeps in quite late most days.

"What have I got to get up to?" Ed asks.

"Well, you could go for a walk ..."

How has their relationship been affected by Ed's dementia?

"I get frustrated, and he gets mad at me."

They smile. They know each other too well.

She's learned much from other caregivers she's met through the Alzheimer's Association.

"What works for one may not work for another, but you try anyway." She's educated herself about sleeping habits and how dementia patients tend to sleep a lot. Medication is often the cause of that. "But it's also their way of getting around reality in some aspects."

Though their children assist them, "I can't count on the kids all the time. It's not fair to them."

What are her limits when asking for help?

"I really don't ask for too much help. If I can't get it done, it doesn't get done. I'm trying to find a handyman. I shouldn't have to expect the kids to come over and do these things, because there's no reason we can't do it, even if it takes us three days to do it."

How do the kids respond?

"They get mad at me." Shirley laughs.

Ed asks, "They get mad at you?"

" 'Why didn't you call, Mom? We would have done it.' " One child became upset when Shirley said she'd hire somebody. She admits she's stubborn. "I think it's from doing so much on our own. Our parents didn't live close by. Everything we did, we did on our own. If we went out, we got a babysitter."

However, she acknowledges that she does worry about Ed, who had fallen and broken his wrist a couple of months earlier.

"After he fell, that was scary. If he had broken more than his wrist, I don't know what I would do." Plus, she worries what will happen to him if something happens to her.

"None of us are infallible from any disease. Your health is in God's hands. When He's ready for you, He's ready for you. The dear Lord will take care of us or help us through our problems."

And what's on the top of the list of Ed's coping skills?

"Faith," he says. "It works."

Adapting to new realities

Expect many changes and challenges in helping a loved one cope with his or her dementia or memory loss. Consider the following new realities:

Food and diet

They may refuse to eat healthy foods or may simply forget to eat or that they had eaten earlier in the day. Consult with their physician, a dietitian or a nutritionist for tips on suitable substitutes or ways to "sneak" healthy items into other foods they're willing to consume. Here are a few suggestions:

▸ *Perhaps there are certain flavors or aromas that will awaken their taste buds. Be willing to experiment.*

▸ *Maybe they won't eat their favorite fruit but will drink it in juice form or vice versa.*

▸ *Maybe they want six small meals a day instead of three bigger ones.*

▸ *Many Alzheimer's individuals "go back in time," so research what their favorite foods were decades ago or when they were growing up. See if there are old family recipes or favorites that they'll like, something their mother or grandmother prepared.*

▸ *Offer portions on a smaller dish if a full plate is too much for them at one sitting.*

▸ *Observe how much liquid they're drinking and if smaller glasses might be easier for them to handle and ease any sensation of being overwhelmed by the amount in the cup.*

▸ *Avoid serving something very hot to drink or eat without allowing it to cool off. They may not remember how hot their favorite coffee or tea is.*

▸ *Don't ask if they want sugar, salt or other condiments. That's one less decision for them to make if you automatically add what they've always taken with their food or beverage.*

▸ *When dining out, they may forget this is their favorite restaurant and what they always ordered. Subtly gesture to the wait staff to take your order first. You'll often find they'll order what you do because the menu overwhelms them, or they may ask what you suggest, so order their favorite. It preserves their dignity.*

Around the house

They may have favorite furniture or objects around the house that give them comfort and security. This isn't the time to introduce new items or rearrange familiar surroundings.

▶ *No matter how weathered or outdated their easy chair is, leave it alone.*

▶ *Keep favorite blankets, pillows or other items out and easy to find.*

▶ *Condense the number of remote controls and stick to the one that is the easiest for them to operate.*

▶ *Keep favorite movies or music out in view for easy access.*

▶ *Keep nearby favorite books, magazines or newspaper. They may not want to read or be able to comprehend the printed words anymore, but they may enjoy looking at photos of favorite activities.*

▶ *Don't be surprised or upset if they go through drawers or closets looking for specific objects. Put things back together and don't expect them to remember exactly what went where.*

Getting to know your loved one again

A loved one with dementia or memory loss will exhibit new behaviors over time, and this will require an adjustment on everyone's part, those who live with this individual and family and friends who are in frequent or sporadic contact.

Use the worksheets on the following four pages to create a new database of information about your loved one as all of you adapt. Have this completed form available for family or friends who offer to stay with your loved one while you take a break or run errands.

Some of the topics may seem unnecessary, but what if your loved one is now inexplicitly angered or scared by something or someone that never bothered them before. Pay attention to those subtle or obvious fluctuations. You can never predict the behavior of someone with Alzheimer's or related conditions.

And be prepared to update this list and add new items as the disease progresses, because the answers — and their interests, tastes and behavior — may change many times.

For the record

What you need to know about me
(the individual with dementia or memory loss)

Diagnosis _____

Physician _____

Phone number _____

Back-up physician to call _____

Phone number _____

Pharmacy _____

Phone number _____

Address _____

Medications _____

Allergies _____

Symptoms to be concerned about _____

Hospital in case of emergency _____

Location of important paperwork _____

I'm good with remembering names _____

I'm not-so-good remembering names _____

Favorite activities _____

Favorite games _____

Favorite foods _____

Favorite snacks _____

Foods I don't like _____

Times I usually eat _____

Food already prepared _____

Favorite beverages _____

Favorite TV show and time it's on _____

Favorite morning show _____

Favorite afternoon show _____

Favorite evening show _____

Favorite weekend show _____

I like watching TV news _____

I can or can't operate the TV by myself _____

Favorite radio show and time it's on _____

I can or can't operate the radio by myself _____

Favorite music, records, tapes, CD's _____

I can or can't operate the player by myself _____

Favorite movies, VHS or DVD _____

I can or can't operate the player by myself _____

People I enjoy seeing _____

People who make me laugh_____

People who upset me _____

Things that upset me _____

People who scare me _____

Things that scare me _____

People who anger me _____

Things that anger me _____

People who calm me _____

114

Things that calm me _____

Noises or sounds that bother me _____

Noises or sounds that I like or calm me _____

I usually lay down for a nap at _____

I rarely take naps _____

Favorite pillow _____

Favorite blanket _____

Favorite piece of furniture _____

Favorite clothes _____

Favorite object _____

Favorite photo _____

Favorite color _____

I have trouble hearing _____

I hear perfectly fine and you don't need to shout _____

I keep misplacing my eyeglasses _____

I like to take walks _____

I like to take car rides _____

I like to go _____

I like to see _____

I like to talk about _____

I don't like to talk about _____

I like to hear jokes _____

I like to hear about _____

I can answer the phone _____

I can't answer the phone _____

I can't take a message _____

My favorite books _____

I can read _____

I can read but like to be read to _____

I can't read any more and like to be read to _____

I read the newspaper every day _____

_____

_____

_____

_____

_____

_____

_____

_____

_____

In her own words

"I'm not afraid of living alone," Wilma announces. "I don't answer the door. No way. I might turn on the porch light to see if it's somebody I know. I feel like I'm safe here as long as I do what I'm supposed to do. My kids don't have to worry about me."

One of her children calls every day. A friend across the street stops by often to check on her.

"It's boring to be alone. It really is. Very boring. If I go outside, I take my keys with me. I never leave my door open. I don't walk very far because if I fall, who will help me?"

Though it's less comfortable being in a large group, she says, "I like to be around people." She had to quit going to a civic group she had belonged to for years, and members stopped calling after a while. Her daughter says her mother looks forward to attending the next support group meeting at the Alzheimer's office.

"We've all got something in common," Wilma says.

What's that?

"Forgetfulness, loneliness." She grins again. "I believe in enjoying myself. I'm not an old fogey."

• • • • •

The 77-year-old woman intently focuses on the paper towel she's been scribbling on for the last five minutes. Delores nods when asked about her diagnosis of Alzheimer's.

"What I want to remember, I seem to remember. Different phone numbers that I always call. I can still pick up the phone and call." She sighs. "I just automatically take (my medicine) in the morning and at night."

Has she talked with her family about what she's thinking about her disease?

"Nobody ever says anything about it. It's kind of like it's a secret."

Is she embarrassed?

"No. I told several people. If they ask, I tell them. People ask, 'What's that?' It means I can't remember."

Everyday realities...

"You've got to do something"

On the drive back to her house after being diagnosed with
Alzheimer's, Sue's mother said, "That doctor's just wrong. I
don't have that." She soon forgot they had seen the doctor.

"I was able to maintain her in her own home for two years
after my father died, but it was bad. It was bad. I would go every
weekend. I noticed she was not eating, but there was food in the
refrigerator there from the week before. I would call every night,
'Now, go take your medicine and come back and tell me.' She'd
tell me she did, but I'd find doses she hadn't taken.

"She was losing a lot of weight. They turned off the cable. I'd
go over and try to help get bills paid. My brother was trying to
help. Mom had a sister who was 86, who also tried to help. She'd
call and say, 'You've got to do something.' Finally, I moved her
into my home for four and a half years, but it got to the point
where we didn't feel comfortable leaving her alone.

"We tried home care, different things. I had a private sitter,
someone I knew, which was my best experience. We also tried a
private duty nurse coming to the house, but Mom would lock
her out because she couldn't remember who she was."

A new job for a couple of years

Peg's husband finally agreed to cut back on his involvement
in the family business when it overwhelmed him. He loved to
play golf, and that was fine most of the year. However, she knew
winter would be difficult. He registered for a class at the local
community college.

Soon he was asked to teach GED classes, Peg explains, which
was perfect because originally, he was a teacher. He did well for
more than two years until he started losing his temper at work,
and that ended his teaching career.

He still drove, even though he often couldn't find his car in
the parking lot. A guard would often drive him around to find
the vehicle. He could then drive home, she remembers.

"Take your special moments, cherish them to the fullest"

Nothing keeps Joe away from his beloved golf course.

"This is a beautiful day. You're not going to waste my time, are you?" Joe asks the visitor.

"No, I wouldn't do anything to keep you off the golf course."

"Terrific!" He laughs.

What else does he like to do?

"I don't know." He turns to his wife Molly. "What do I like to do, honey?"

"Golf. You like watching old movies over and over again."

"Sure do."

"The classic statement you made one day, Joe, when the doctor said, 'You're here because of memory loss?' You said, 'That's what they say.' It's hard to know you have memory loss, because if it's gone, how do you know you've lost it? It's other people who tell you. It's not a conspiracy, nothing we're plotting, just the things we've noticed. The kids have noticed it, too. That's how it all started."

More than three years ago, Molly's suspicions were aroused when she noticed that his checkbook wasn't balanced. That was very unusual because Joe had been in sales and kept detailed records. The other clue was how names were beginning to escape him. Names wouldn't stick on people he had known the least amount of time.

"Joe and I needed to be sure about things. First, we went to our attorney and made sure all our papers were in order. We wanted to do it at a time when Joe could participate because the time may come when he can't.

"Our family doctor asked him a lot of questions. She said, 'Yep, memory loss.' I don't know if it was hope against all hope, but I thought I saw a change (with the medication). I thought I saw the cloud being moved, the sun rising."

She looks at him.

"My mouth gets dry after a while. I need for you to jump in here, Buddy."

Everyone laughs.

"I thought, 'The doctor has got this right on.' Then the quiet came in and that started to bother me. All the while, I'm going to the Alzheimer's Association office for education. We make another trip back to the doctor, and I told her about the quietness, and that's when she introduced you to another drug. Once again, I saw this great change. I was getting sentences, and the humor seemed to be back. I don't know if it was really there, or me wishing it was."

Referred to another physician, Joe underwent extensive tests. "The sweetest, dearest thing came out of that testing session. As we were leaving after talking to the doctor, a nurse came running out of the office with a sheet of paper. She said, 'Look at this. All patients have to write a sentence, and Joe wrote, 'I love my wife.'

"Oh, look at you sitting there," she admonishes her smiling husband. "She said, 'This doesn't happen. These are not the sentences we're used to getting.' That was a very charming, wonderful thing. You scored points there, Buddy. I knew you meant it. Indeed. It's hard to tell with Joe. Look at him. He's got that look on his face right now."

"I don't know what to say," he says. "You covered it so well."

"Do you remember that?" Molly asks.

"I remember most of it, yes."

"After the CT scan, the doctor said there were no stroke signs, but your brain was getting smaller, and that is a sign of Alzheimer's. So, that's what we're dealing with. You're not sure which pills you take now, are you?"

"I'm not sure." He shakes his head.

"You take a bunch of them. This getting old is not an easy thing to do. Then your eyes start going, and you can't count them out." She smiles. "Joe takes naps with an 80-pound dog. She's a true delight."

"Yes, she is."

"What do you call her?"

"What do we call her?"

"You know her name."

"Oh, uh …" He's thinking.

"You go to the door and call her all the time. What's her name?"

"Of course. I do it all the time."

"Go call her. You'll remember that way."

Laughing, he shakes his finger again to free that memory. What color is she?

"She's brownish. She's a very, very good dog. We're lucky."

"What's her name?"

"Mattie." He smiles in triumph.

The visitor asks how many children they have.

"We've got ..." He pauses in thought. "How many kids do we have? We have ... Don't tell me." He points at her.

"I'm not going to," Molly says.

"I know they come here quite often."

See, his memory isn't *that* bad.

Molly gives him a hint. "Our oldest lives in Wisconsin."

"Our oldest lives in Wisconsin. In Wisconsin? John."

"Who's the child after John?"

"That would be Tom."

"And there's a child after Tom. A beautiful child. Sometimes known as your precious baby."

"She's a beauty. Uh ... I know her name. I just ..."

"You're going on a trip with her."

"I am?"

"Yes. What's your daughter's name?" Silence. "She teaches hearing impaired children."

"She does. She sure does."

"What's her name?"

"I can't think of it."

The pain glistens in Molly's eyes.

"Oh my God," she whispers. "It starts with an M."

Silence.

"Yeah, I do know this ... I ... I know their names. I know who they are. Why, somehow I just can't seem to ..."

"John, Tom and who?" Molly asks.

"John?"

"Tom and who?" Molly asks again.

"And ... John, Tom and ... What's the girl's name?"

Silence.

Molly reassures him. "I know it will come to you. I'm not going to tell you."

"Good."

"It will come to you. It will come to you very soon."

"Yeah."

T hat's the killer of this thing," Molly says. "Every day is different. This is not a repeat of Groundhog's Day. This is, right now, a rough morning. This proves it. But tomorrow morning, it may not be like this. That's the strange thing about this. Doctors can make a diagnosis on what they see. They will put a person in a certain category. But the one who really knows the person can read these different requirements and categories and can say, 'Not there, here, but not this, here.' It jumps around, and it's not always consistent. Because Joe knows the name of his daughter. I know he knows the name of his daughter."

He says a name.

"No, that's one of your grandchildren. Margy is not married. Margy has no children. Oh, geez!"

Molly throws her hands up. She's given it away, but has he caught it? Laughter erupts despite this sad moment.

"Wait a minute," he says. "Let me think. Margy comes ..."

"What Margy's long name?"

"Margaret Mary, I don't know."

"Yes, it is!"

"Right." He's pleased.

Shaking her head, she can't avoid the smile.

"You look to me all the time when you're stuck because you want me to talk for you."

"Yes, of course, I'm sure I would. That wouldn't surprise me."

That's what wives are for, the visitor jokes.

"That's exactly what they're for," he announces.

Everyone laughs.

"Okay, now, I know my place," she says.

He relies a lot on Molly, doesn't he?

"Oh, yes. Yes, I do."

Does she take good care of him?

"Oh, yes."

Molly asks, "What's something I could do better for you?"

"You know what? When I think back, I think you're flawless."

"Yes, but that's thinking back," she teases. "That may have changed. What do you think now?"

"I mean it."

"What do you think right now?"

"About what?"

"Am I helping you?"

"How do you mean?"

"Am I helping you daily?"

"I think I would easily say yes. Definitely."

"We wear our bracelets faithfully, don't we?"

"Yep, we do."

"Why are you wearing that bracelet? Do you remember who put that on you?"

"You did."

"No. Your daughter did. What's her name?"

There's a long pause.

"Margy?"

"Do you remember what she said when she put that on you?"

"No." He studies the bracelet.

"Why did she want you to wear that?"

"I don't know."

"I wear one, too. Why am I wearing one?"

"You're doing it for the same reason?"

"Yes."

"Hmm …"

"You're not sure why?"

"I can't say that I do."

"Can you think of any reason why we would both be wearing the same bracelet?"

"Well, I'm pretty sure why now." His jaw tightens.

"You don't remember what Margy said when she gave it to you?"

"No. What did she say?"

"She said, 'I want you to keep this on always. In case something happens to Mom, they'll know there's a you because we're both wearing the same number. Or if anything happens to you, you can show somebody your bracelet, and they can find us, get us together. That's why it's important.'

"If I were in a car accident," Molly says, "and unable to talk, a doctor could see this and they'd know by reading the back that I'm your caregiver, and they're going to find you so you're not left alone. Otherwise they won't know. The same thing goes for you. If something happens to you, they can find me. It makes sense, doesn't it?"

"Yes, it does."

The visitor asks if this means they're going steady again?

"Are we?" Joe grins.

Molly laughs and returns to the bracelet.

"It's a Safe Return bracelet. It's a very important to wear."

"Safe Return, huh?"

"Do you see that design on the front?"

"What is it?"

"A path."

"A path?"

123

"See the path?"

"It's got a lot of information on it."

"What does it say?"

"It's kind of hard to look at." He studies it. "Can you read it? Don't you have it?"

"Yes, I have it."

"I can't quite make it out."

"There are two numbers, a phone number, and an identification number. It's a good thing to wear, isn't it?"

"Yes, it is."

Molly pauses. "Now I will tell you a funny story. Yesterday, I put soup in the crockpot and went to work. When I got home, it smelled so good. Well, this morning, when we got back from the gym, I could still smell the soup. So, I gave Joe a bottle of air refresher and said, 'Will you run around the house and do some spraying?' Joe literally ran through the house spraying. You said, 'Ask me to do anything else, I'll be happy to.' Right?"

"Yes."

"Oh, Joe, sometimes you really make me laugh." She turns to the visitor. "The message is to take your special moments, cherish them to the fullest, and just be sure and get your rest, because it does make you tired. I found out there's nothing wrong with going to bed at 8 o'clock, nothing wrong with a nap. You need to recharge your own batteries if you're a caregiver."

What's been the emotional and physical toll on her so far?

"Worry … about the future. That's something that would loom over anybody's head, not just me. The unknown, and even through the studying I've done and the classes I've taken, there is a path that Alzheimer's takes … that I hope God would spare us, because that final stage … has to be hard. When we talk to God, we ask Him to lighten our load. These are supposed to be the good years ... the 'Golden Years' they call them, and they're hard. And it's okay to cry, to show emotion. It's okay to sit in silence, too. Right, Joe?"

"Right, Molly."

As his eyes fill with tears, he glances away.

"That's the part of love that hurts when you see someone who used to be extremely outgoing person, funny, funny person ... When you see that being destroyed, you develop a hatred of the disease because of what it does and how it affects people.

"Granted, now it has a name. When I was a kid, a person who was old had hardening of the arteries, a little dementia. Now, it's being put into categories, and there are so many categories for dementia and yet, we are not positive that you, Joe, have Alzheimer's. The only way to tell is at death ... So you take these learned men and women in their infinite wisdom and I guess you place your trust in them. You put all the faith you have in God and say, 'Help me through this.' "

Her daughter plans to take Joe on a three-day vacation, which will allow her "to refresh my soul and body a little bit, which is wonderful. They're great children, aren't they, Joe?"

"Yes, they are, dear, very good."

She encourages every one to get to their local Alzheimer's Association office for help immediately.

During her first visit, she admits, "I was scared to death. I think initially when it hits you, you feel so alone and that no one will understand, that it is a shameful thing, not shameful, but degrading. 'This can't be happening to me and my family.' Then you find out there are so many people out there that it's affecting.

"When you start talking in the group, someone will say, 'Oh, yeah, ... does that' or 'I haven't noticed that.' It's like a spider web with so many different paths to take." She tells of a friend who passes along information to a family in an area where an Alzheimer's Association is not nearby.

"There is power in knowledge. When the doctor diagnosed Joe and put him in a certain category, I started reading these categories and said, 'No, he's not there. You don't see this. Maybe in the office, he appeared that way to you, but it's not true.' That's where this power comes from, and you say, 'No, he's not there. Yeah, maybe two out of the 10 characteristics are present, but the other eight aren't.' There is no complete niche where everybody goes."

The visitor turns to Joe and says, "You're unique ... in more ways than one."

"Good. I was hoping someone would say I was unique."

"Joe, you are unique," Molly says.

"I didn't want to say anything myself, you know what I mean." He chuckles.

Molly laughs. "I know. What are your kids' names, Joe?"

"We went through all that already."

Yes, forever the jokester.

"People may not admit Alzheimer's nor recognize it, but I know it's there." She looks at Joe. "You agree, don't you, Buddy?"

"I agree."

"I know you do, Buddy. One nice thing about you, Joe, you're always on my side."

"I disagree with that."

He laughs the loudest.

Molly gives up.

"That's kind of how my day goes. There are times when I totally crack up and times I cry ..."

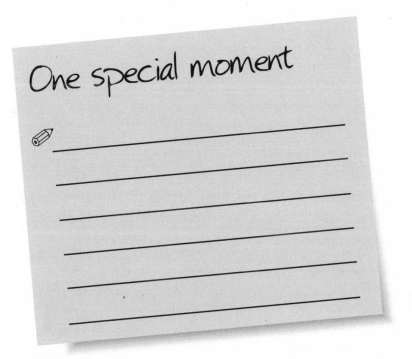

One special moment

Just talking...

(Caregiver and client responses and reactions are in italics.)

Another winter fades into memory, and spring offers new challenges and a desire to learn for about a dozen pairs of recently diagnosed clients and their immediate caregivers. Some faces are familiar and others are new to the educational and support group format.

Many of the life issues are still the same, yet bear repeating ... especially for those who cannot remember ...

It's not a pleasant subject, but a very necessary one, says Jenn, facilitating this portion of the meeting. It's time to address the issues of power of attorney, wills, long-term care, etc.

"Don't make important decisions in a crisis," she advises.

Caregivers need to plan ahead if something does happen to them first because the patient won't be able to make those decisions. Carry that information in the car, on your person and in the client's wallet or purse. Create a "what-if" list.

During the breakout session with the caregivers, Bonnie continues that subject with the following observations:

▸ *Individuals often do well and actually better in an adult day care setting, which is more stimulating than being at home. Then the family thinks they should bring them home, when it's being at the day care that is assisting them.*

▸ *Don't wipe out your financial options.*

▸ *If necessary, research the eligibility for Medicaid beds and make the right choice for your situation. Nursing facilities generally request six months to two years of private pay, though some may have sliding scale.*

▸ *There's a waiting and priority list for beds, a compilation that is "longer than any of us will live in some cases."*

▸ *Think about your options ahead of time. Being prepared is the best decision.*

Families have to ask themselves the importance of decisions because there's an upside and downside to any choice. What is the philosophy of the adult day care center or nursing home? What environment will be able to handle the changing capabilities of your loved one? Do an unannounced drop-in visit, and remember that the care is only as good as the staff that shows up, she adds.

A lso remember that there is no perfect place and that accidents can happen anywhere, even in the home. Bonnie asks if all of them have turned down the temperature on their hot water heater because clients may not realize just how hot it is and are burned.

127

"I'd better make a note for the family meeting."

One caregiver toured an adult day care and discovered that some of the attendees act as volunteers, which helps them feel better and that they're making a contribution.

Your attitude is a huge factor in how people respond to you, Bonnie explains. The way you treat the staff can have a direct effect on how they treat your loved one. Thank them for anything and everything. Thank the cleaning persons.

"A little bit of sugar goes a long way."

Make a "feel good folder" with notes and cartoons in it that will help carry you through a tough time, she says.

One husband is doing work for a neighbor.

One caregiver laments that some places have the audacity to call themselves self-care.

Bonnie reminds them of the need to look at the full story. Every place will be the right place for someone.

"I wanted to bring my brother home with me, but my husband said our schedule wouldn't match his."

Bonnie says that we can all say that we don't want our loved ones in assisted living or a nursing home, but they often do much better. They're never by themselves, they get their meds on time, and most importantly, they eat properly.

"The upside of dementia is that they won't remember you promised. You should only say that 'I'll do my very best to keep you safe.' It's an issue of keeping them and you safe. If you can't, then that's what you have to do. It's far worse if someone gets hurt because you didn't do the right thing."

It's easy to make a promise in the beginning.

"We all have an idea of what we hope will happen, but it's too much out of our control. Know that you made the best decision you could make that day."

"We are vitally important to our people."

It's a fine line of knowing the right time. Is he or she going to wander onto the highway? Caregivers need to know what to do for themselves.

"He said to 'do what is best for you.' "

It's hard to move them from one type of care or one facility to another after becoming accustomed to the staff and place overall. Besides, you hate change, too, Bonnie adds.

One session focuses on how families can partner with their physicians to make sure the relationship is mutually beneficial and educational. Alzheimer's Association facilitators Jenn and Chris offer the following reminders.

▸ *Doctors rely on patients and caregivers to provide vital information to provide the best possible care.*

▸ *Individuals with dementia or memory loss need a third party — a caregiver— to be in an equal partnership with the physician and patient.*

▸ *It's often a long time between appointments, so plan for visits and write down questions that may come up along the way.*

▸ *Keep a log of how the patient is doing, such as sleeping and eating habits or behavior that might indicate pain that the patient can't clearly articulate.*

▸ *Symptoms or behavior that we may think are not important may be vital in helping the doctor pinpoint problems not associated with the dementia or memory loss.*

▸ *Ask yourself, "Do I understand all topics brought up during this appointment?" Tell the doctor, "Let me make sure I understand ..."*

▸ *Review highlights of the visit with others involved in caregiving.*

A caregiver says the visits can be stressful, and it's easy to forget pertinent information like medications and dosages patients are currently taking. She makes sure she takes in a written list of all prescription and over-the-counter medicines.

That is important information to provide all physicians a patient may see because some medicine combinations can be harmful or cancel out the effectiveness of another.

Another says the doctor asks if they have any questions, and some-times the caregiver is too afraid to ask or may have 1,000 inquiries. It's hard to cram in so much in so little time.

"When the doctor said to take it one day at a time, I knew I was in trouble," another caregiver says with a smile.

"If we're organized," suggests another, "then they have more time to doctor."

Jenn and Chris advise them to not feel like victims and speak up. Though there are some doctors with poor bedside manners, that is not an excuse to ignore asking the important questions related to the well-being of your loved one.

129

As the caregivers meet, they discuss their latest challenges …

One client walks to the end of the hallway at home and is exhausted. Another has forgotten where dishes go.

"Mom's afraid of water now."

One is in a power struggle over proper eating habits with their loved one, who's losing too much weight.

One husband is starting to just sit in his chair for 10-12 hours a day and won't do anything else.

"It's scary, wondering every day what else is going to happen."

A mother says her son told her she was not putting his father in a nursing home, no matter what. She says he just doesn't understand what caring for his father every day has done and will do to her.

Another laments that she didn't notice the signs earlier, and every-one tells her not to feel guilty because it's so gradual. They understand what she's going through.

"I find the shower is the greatest place to cry …"

Where's my escape?

_____

_____

_____

_____

_____

Caregivers say...

As noted earlier, we all respond and cope differently to stressful situations, especially after a devastating diagnosis of a loved one's Alzheimer's, dementia or memory loss. Everyone derives strength from different sources or seeks refuge from reality in things that can help us forget our worries and frustrations ... at least for a while.

What things helped you cope or thrive?

▸ Help from siblings

▸ Support group

▸ Educational video tapes

▸ Attending programs at the Alzheimer's Association

▸ Alzheimer's Web site

▸ Relatives living nearby

▸ Hobbies

▸ Help from children

▸ Friends

▸ Caring for other family members

▸ Cards from friends

▸ Notes from family

▸ Online support group

▸ Visiting nurses

▸ Private inner group

▸ Making gifts for veterans' hospital

▸ Love and commitment

▸ I got much help from my brother. We divided tasks. I handled medical and financial, and he handled getting the house ready to be sold and other things. *Kevin, 45, mother, Alzheimer's*

"I had no choice. I did what I had to do until I couldn't anymore, and then he went to a care center." Roseann, 72, husband, dementia, died 10 years after diagnosed

▸ The doctor who gave us the diagnosis and his office help who said call anytime. Also our pastor and church family, my family and friends. *Maxine, 77, husband, Alzheimer's*

- Locating a good quality facility that focused on dementia care, quality care. Being a nurse whose area of expertise is gerontology with a focus on Alzheimer's. *Ann, 49, mother, vascular dementia, died; father, Alzheimer's, died*

- Love was the most important motivation, but without help, I can't do it. *Christl, 55, father, stroke and Alzheimer's*

- My wife and I split the duty, making sure we have personal time. *John, 67, mother-in-law, Alzheimer's*

131

- Knowing that we have been blessed to have him be mentally astute up to age 89. *Mary Ann, 62, father, Alzheimer's*

- Remembering that she once helped me live with dignity when I was a child. *Elizabeth, 47, mother, Alzheimer's*

- Knowing my mother was in a safe and caring place. The workers were very good to her and me at the nursing home. *Jolene, 66, mother, dementia, died 5 years after diagnosed*

- You have to live. That means work, chores and play, and this just happens to be a part. *David, 69, wife, Alzheimer's*

- Yes, knowing I could give Mom peace of mind and a better quality of life with us. She had a hard life. She deserves this care now in her life. *Jenny, 56, mother, Alzheimer's*

- Private counseling and a great boss who let my husband come to work with me. *Sandy, 61, husband, Alzheimer's and vascular dementia*

- The caring staff at the nursing home and understanding the doctors. *Nancy, 65, mother, Alzheimer's*

- I wasn't FROG (Fully Rely On God). So each time I saw my frog watch or stuffed animal, it reminded me I wasn't alone in this. An adult day care center was a big help. *MM, 46, mother, Alzheimer's, died 5 years after diagnosed*

"My children, they filled the freezer, precooked meals, gave me 'time off' and helped financially." *Anne, 67, mother, dementia, died 4 years after diagnosed*

"We're affected by all this but you aren't — why?"

At age 22, Matt should have entered the "real world" to make it on his own. Instead, he was pre-occupied with the altered reality of his father, diagnosed at age 51 with dementia.

"I'm kind of having to be the parent. My whole life, him being there and doing everything for me … and then all of a sudden, the role switches.

"I was very close to my dad." Matt describes the relationship he and his older brother had with him. "He was always there coaching, teaching us. He was the person, when you want to stay out late or do something, you'd go to your dad instead of your mom." He laughs. "He was a laid-back, fun-loving person.

"Dad was a sales person all his life, very outgoing, friendly. At work, when he was 49 or 50, he started acting very weird. At meetings, he'd fall asleep and act disinterested. We knew it wasn't him, but we couldn't pinpoint what the problem was."

Due to the erratic behavior, he lost his job. He showed little emotion for anyone except himself, which wasn't like him at all. Matt had noticed his failing memory. For example, Matt talked about long-ago trips, but his dad couldn't come up with any specifics, only, "Yeah, I remember." But he didn't.

"It was really hard on me that I had all these great times, and he was forgetting it all. *'What's your problem? What's happening?'* He thought everything was fine in his head." He became a compulsive eater, and it was increasingly hard to take him out. "He'd make weird comments to strangers, not have the social norms. It was tough having to 'baby-sit' him in social situations. At dinners, he'd grab people's plates. *'Why are you eating so much? Why are you doing that?' 'I'm fine.'* It was embarrassing."

Eventually, Matt says, they had to lock the kitchen cabinets. However, he unscrewed the doors, so they had to hide the screwdrivers. They taped the refrigerator shut at night. He'd sneak down later and tear the tape off. It became a sad game as the family would catch him in the act and end up chasing him playfully.

How did the son's feelings evolve over time? In the beginning, he was angry with his father's eating habits and behavior because the family didn't know the source of his problem. "We're all affected by this, but you aren't. Why?" It became easier to not take him anywhere. "Why set him up for failure?

"At Christmas, we were at a relatives' home, and the little girls had put cookies out for Santa, and my dad ate all the cookies!" He laughs now at the uncomfortable memory. "My aunt was really mad. This was before the diagnosis. She was making snide comments, and I said I ate some of them to cover for him."

Finally, after extensive testing, during which everything from depression to early-onset Alzheimer's was considered the possible cause, it was finally labeled as frontal lobe dementia.

"Once I knew what it was, it was a relief. This is the reason he's acting this way. It's not a weird mid-life crisis, he really has a bad disease. It's affecting his reasoning and social behavior." Anger eased into understanding, though it's devastating to learn about this fatal disease.

"What do they know about my dad? He should be living forever. To put an expiration date on his life … you can't imagine that."

While his mother continued to work, the family hired someone to watch him during the day. However, after he shoved this person to get more food, they faced difficult decisions as he couldn't stay at home any longer. Their best option was a healthcare center that worked with Alzheimer's patients, and Matt remembers some of the facilities' employees were amazed at how long he had remained at home.

It's not been an easy journey for the mother and two sons, who witnessed this horrible deterioration of the man they loved. The stress mounted for all of them, but he now understands how every family has to make its own decisions in providing care.

"All these things you take for granted are taken away. I think my mom has gotten a lot of strength from my brother and me, because we're a lot like our dad. We get a lot from her." However, his mom's lifelong partner is "gone" now. She's alone. "It's going to be so much bigger for her than for us. I need to be less selfish and take care of her."

While away at college, he's witnessed huge changes in his dad between visits. When it finally clicks with his father after 10 to 15 minutes who he is, Matt jokes with him.

"He doesn't have to say words, but it's just real tough to see him in a really bad situation from what he used to be. It's not something I could deal with every single day. You can leave and live your life. We don't have to worry about the daily aspects of his everyday life. My mom is getting used to letting him go …

"My best way of coping, though not a good way, is not really dealing with it. I've enjoyed being away at school because I don't want to see my dad this way. It's horrible. I want to see him, but that blank look in his eyes and how it takes 10 minutes for him to remember me, is really tough. I like to think of the good memories.

"I look at my brother like my dad now, because my dad's there, but he's not." The young man's voice shakes. "My older brother has always been there for me and will continue to be there. I have a much better relationship with him, and it's been strengthened (by this). He's a good fatherly influence."

He pauses. "Sometimes, I'll just break down and cry because I haven't gotten it out in the proper way." He's saddened and jealous when he sees fathers and sons his age together and enjoying each other. He doesn't have that anymore. He says his mom wanted him to talk to a counselor, but he refused.

"I don't want to sit down with a stranger and just spout. My mom is in support groups. She gets a lot of strength listening to their stories." However, support groups aren't for him at this point. He's just someone who doesn't ask for help. He admits he found himself drinking more alcohol, but that only masked the problem for a short time.

"I'm a selfish person, and I'm always thinking about what I wanted to do." He'd go out with friends and come home late or the next morning, and it made the situation worse because his mother would blow up at him for his behavior, especially if he had been drinking. "It's opened my eyes and how I need to think of other's people's needs." That's been a gradual internal change.

It's also awakened him to a new dimension of human behavior. Few friends knew what was occurring, but people knew something was amiss.

"You find out who your real friends are when times aren't good. It's as simple as asking a person, 'Hey, how's your dad doing?' Just one sentence, just one show of empathy goes so far. I realized who my parents' friends were and who tried to help out and cared about the situation. Just keeping up-to-date with it, compared to avoiding it."

At the same time, Matt believes most of it stems from people simply not knowing what to do or say. He isn't sure how he would have reacted toward a friend going through the same experience. He remembers a high school friend whose mother died from cancer, and he admits he didn't know what to say or do even though he went to the funeral.

"You feel isolated when you're in the situation and people are out there not doing anything. They don't know what to do or what's right."

What does he want people to say and do for him?

"Just acknowledge that the situation exists. I'm not expecting anybody to do anything special. Just because he's in a home now, real friends could visit." He acknowledges that it's awkward to bring it up. " *'How's this sick person doing?'* It's tough to do. I think it's human nature to avoid problems and concerns. It's more comfortable to stay on the good stuff, not the bad stuff."

He wanted to slug a friend who didn't talk to his own parents.

"He treats them like crap. I never said anything to him, but I wanted to say, *'You have no idea what you're missing. You never know what tomorrow will bring.'* I had a very easy childhood. This was the first big hurdle in my life. How do you respond to that? My family and I have done a great job getting through this."

Does he resent any of the sacrifices he's made so far in coping with his father's illness?

"It's the future I'm sad about, for what I won't be able to experience with him … being at my wedding or becoming a grandparent."

While his dad exists in his own little world, Matt faces his own challenges and worries. His mother's brother was diagnosed with Alzheimer's, and his grandmother had it. The latter was particularly sad because she had always been nice and loving but became mean and said horrible things.

Is he worried about it affecting him? He jokes with his brother, " *'Me or you?'* If I have an expiration date of age 50, I'm going to enjoy life."

What would his dad tell him now to help? He smiles.

"He'd make a joke out of it. I know that for a fact. He'd rely on humor to get through all these situations in life."

Just talking...

(Caregiver and client responses and reactions are in italics.)

As the educational and support group for recently diagnosed clients and their immediate caregivers reconvenes, a participant asks when someone with dementia or memory loss can't or shouldn't drive anymore.

A voice rings out, "When you hit a few people."

Like a child who says the cutest, yet most inappropriate, thing, everyone can't help but laugh. Her comment definitely breaks the ice on a delicate topic.

Another laments that "I passed everything, but they wrote 'no driving.'" Next to her, her daughter just smiles and shakes her head.

Bonnie, one of the facilitators, takes this cue to explain how perception, vision and reaction time are affected by dementia and memory loss. The memory we rely on to automatically respond to driving challenges can fail unexpectedly, leaving the driver unsure how to respond in a situation. Plus, the driver may not be paying attention to other cars or pedestrians because of the memory shortfalls. Depth perception is crucial in driving, and that ability is hampered by changes in the brain.

One client suggests that the doctor say no to driving to avoid potential lawsuits. Nods sweep the room.

A client, a former driving instructor, says he saw many women who had to learn to drive later in life because of their husband's inability to take the wheel anymore.

Bonnie adds that some families continue to let memory loss individuals drive mostly for convenience. The end of driving is a huge loss to a person.

One husband says he's not allowed to drive without his wife.

Another adds, "They won't even let me do that."

A woman recalls her first driving experience, stepping on the gas at about age 8 and ending up in the middle of the street. "A few police officers rescued me."

"Your mom is a juvenile offender, and you didn't even know it," someone tells the woman's laughing daughter.

A client says it bothers him that he can't drive, and his wife notes, "Our friends worry about him when they see him walking down a busy street to go shopping."

He turns to her and says, "Can I explain?" In silence, she nods and looks down as he tells how a friend yelled at him to get in the car. "It gets old walking on the same path."

"I have to ask," says another. "I can't go anywhere I want."

At this moment around the big circle of individuals united by dementia or memory loss, it becomes obvious that this frustration is shared.

Bonnie interjects some of the realities of clients driving. Loved ones often fear the clients will get lost because one wrong turn can throw them off completely. That happens to everybody occasionally when roads suddenly don't look familiar, but with memory loss, it could be 100 miles out of their way, and self-correcting is harder or even impossible without assistance. It's easy to get lost driving places they've gone for years.

The conversation about cars continues for the clients with facilitators Jenn and Alisha after the caregivers leave the room. Alisha asks if they prefer manual or automatic transmission.

"It doesn't make a difference. I'll wreck them all."

"I love manual and love to drive, but they won't let me."

"I'm going to get a horse."

This session is a great conversation starter for the men who start spouting off specifics about engines and car styles.

"They won't let me drive anymore because I have dementia."

Alisha asks, "How do you feel?"

"I find somebody to go with me. I respect their decision for safety. I can drive if my wife goes with me."

Another is mad at "that crazy doctor. I never in my life had a ticket."

Alisha asks a client who told him he had to quit driving.

"You'd think I'd remember." He shrugs and smiles. "Dementia."

The caregivers share their own driving stories with Bonnie … *One husband drove when he was not supposed to. He told her that he thought he was missing coffee with his buddies. She told him he hadn't thought of the consequences. Luckily she's kept their car insurance in force for him if something happens.*

Bonnie explains that it was his instinct and the dementia that created that situation.

Another says her husband took off to drive for the first time in five years. She was a nervous wreck and called 911.

One spouse wants to drive but can't because of medication.

One tells of how her loved one took her driving test and nearly hit a woman. The individual used Alzheimer's as an excuse and then was flunked only after saying that.

For others facing similar circumstances, Bonnie suggests the doctor write the prescription denying the license.

A caregiver recommends calling the driver's license branch ahead of time to tell them to turn down their loved one.

Taking away the car keys

Vicky remembers the day her husband, Tom, who had early-onset Alzheimer's, went out shopping and didn't come home. They finally reached him on his cell phone, and he returned after 10:30 p.m. Their daughter felt terrible for telling him where to go shopping out of town.

She paid more attention to his driving, and after a couple of close calls, she decided to take away the keys. At the same time, he got a speeding ticket, and she asked his doctor to fill out forms to remove his license. She wouldn't be able to ever forgive herself if something happened to him or someone else.

He got a letter from the state reporting that his driver's license had been revoked. He was upset, unaware of what they had done.

"The speeding ticket was a blessing in disguise. We blamed it on the 'state,' because it's not someone you can call up and yell at." She told him they couldn't fight the state, and he was irate for hours. "The next day, he was fine. We were blaming the 'big bad state.' "

For Father's Day, their children bought Tom a bicycle and helmet, and he rode that everywhere. He never asked to drive again because it gave him independence. His ability to keep working at a flower shop helped because he was still able to contribute ...

Peg finally had to put an end to her husband's driving by lying about how much she wanted to drive. Two months before she had to take him to a nursing home, he lost his temper and drove away in his truck. She searched everywhere until she finally got a call from someone 30 miles away. Their son and granddaughter picked him up.

"Getting rid of his truck was pure hell, I tell you, pure hell." The family made up a story about their other son in a neighboring city needing it. They drove it away that day, no problem. The next day he remembered nothing about giving them the truck, and he began ranting. By then, "his personality was really bad, really, really bad." Looking back, she doesn't know what she would have done differently …

Jim says they were afraid of his mother driving because she'd only go a short distance and be gone for hours. "She wasn't going to let anyone take the keys from her. She would get lost, even driving a few miles to church." They had to take the keys, while reassuring her that it was okay to get some help …

June recalls, "We had arguments, and I had to use trickery or deceit to do things, like hide the car keys …"

"My mother stopped driving on her own," Sue says, "I think because she kept getting lost. We just quickly got rid of the car."

How we'll take the keys

Educating the public

"He's not deaf"

Molly often uses the card the Alzheimer's Association gave her, which states that this person has trouble with memory loss and how their patience is appreciated.

"I've done some very interesting studies on this. Do you know what happens? The minute you hand it to someone, they assume that person is deaf. They suddenly start talking much louder and say, 'SIR, DO YOU KNOW WHAT YOU WANT TO EAT?' Finally I say, 'He's not deaf.' But isn't that funny?

"One day, I handed the waiter the card, and that waiter immediately got down on his knee so that he was face-to-face with Joe. I asked, 'How did you know to do that?' He said, 'My grandmother …' So, now I'm thinking there is a whole new school of people out there that need to be informed about memory loss and people coming into their place of business. They will start shouting at you, and they even do it in a doctor's office."

"Quit preaching to everyone"

After her husband was diagnosed, Vicky had to explain to people the differences between early-onset, which he had, and the early stages of Alzheimer's. People often don't understand the difference. She's had to explain to people that older individuals have early stages, not early-onset.

"Then I catch myself. This person doesn't need an education. Quit preaching to everyone." She laughs. How does she explain it? Early-onset is a diagnosis if under 60 and geriatric if over 60. If they act interested, she'll explain more.

Making adjustments

"I told my mom that she and I would get through it together until the end. My resolve was set early on." MM, 46, mother, Alzheimer's, died 5 years after diagnosed

In his own words

"Are you going to ask me questions to see if my memory is working?" John laughs.

Despite vascular dementia, his memory has not failed him when it comes to recalling his date of birth, high school graduation, entering the U.S. Navy, various jobs, and the details of meeting his wife, Bev, and their wedding day. Very smart man.

"I realize what's happening," he says. "I'm racking my brain trying to remember simple things. Sometimes I can remember for three seconds and have to ask again and again. But I knew you were coming, and I checked my little note. That's been a struggle all day trying to come up with the name."

However, he claims it doesn't bother him a lot.

"Honestly, you can't get me lost driving because I go with the location of the sun and the compass. In my mind, I know which way is east or west. I know that I would find something familiar. It may take me all day, but I'd find my way home. I think I have fewer problems on an interstate system than in a neighborhood."

He explains that he follows signs and landmarks.

"I love to talk to people I don't know. I wouldn't hesitate to get directions because I'm that kind of person."

How does he think Bev and the rest of family have been affected by his dementia?

"I don't really have …" He pauses and laughs. "I forget the question. I had it my mind how I was going to explain but it's gone." The question is repeated. "It's scary for her, I'm sure. She's doing things, putting a lot of the load on her shoulders. She knows I forget to do this and that. The hardship is on her far more than it is on me. I try real hard to keep our communication on top. We're getting along. I hope I don't get any worse."

John looks at his visitor.

"Is it possible or likely I could lose my memory further on?"

"I don't know" is the only possible response.

"I don't know either."

Nobody knows.

"I'm hoping … if I'm going to lose memory, I hope it's real slow. I hope it just doesn't shut the curtain on me all the way."

"See what all he used to be able to do?"

John and Bev try unsuccessfully to get a living room recliner back to stay in place.

"I'll take it apart," he volunteers.

"No. I don't let him take anything apart," she says. Everyone laughs.

What did she first notice about John's dementia?

"He couldn't learn things." He had a new job but couldn't remember simple tasks, how or what he did. Plus, he kept repeating the same questions. On his hospital bed after open-heart surgery, he was notified he had lost his job.

"He had trouble remembering the grandkids' names." His short-term memory seemed to have eroded. Finally, he went to the doctor and was diagnosed with vascular dementia.

It might get worse or it may not. He may remain at this stage for a long time. They don't know. She says he can't even remember where things go in the cupboard.

John says, "I started blaming Bev. Why would you put the peanut butter here and the jelly there?" She explains every time that one is kept cold and the other doesn't need to be refrigerated.

When asked about the sharing of responsibilities, how this has affected their relationship and how they communicate, John asks with a smile, "That's what I want to know."

Bev says she's taken care of the checkbook for years. "I give him things I think he can do. He does the dishes, runs the sweeper, mows the yard." She gives him specific assignments but can't combine them, such as getting the newspaper and the mail at the same time. "I just try to give him one thing at a time, and he gets his exercise."

"Do you think we work well together?" he asks.

"Yes, you just need some supervision at times." She explains that he easily gets sidetracked on tasks and moves on to something else.

How have their children and grandchildren responded?

"I don't think they recognize the problem," John says.

"Yes, definitely, they do," Bev says, smiling.

"Do they?" He looks surprised.

"They always say, 'Oh, Grandpa, you'll forget that.' " She says he's better one-on-one with the six grandchildren.

What other adjustments have they made? Though they don't want their son to feel obligated, he has taken over major chores around the house they built. Bev gestures at the spacious room.

"See what all John used to be able to do? Now he can hardly work on his tractors anymore." That's why she's not going to let him tinker with the chair.

"I could fix that," he offers again.

"I know you probably could, but you may forget how to put it back together again." She smiles.

He got lost once while they were in Massachusetts. He was gone most of the day and without the phone number where they were staying.

"It was terrifying," he recalls. "I didn't know which way to go. I was always a person who would go anywhere in the country."

"I'm the navigator, but he does the driving," she says. Sometimes he does forget where they are.

"Some days, I think some things just don't click. I get mad at myself."

"Yes, sometimes he gets mad at himself because he can't remember, frustrated with himself."

His mother had Alzheimer's. They didn't recognize the changes in her for a long time.

"She was the nicest person I ever knew, my mother." He sits back sad. "At the nursing home, she had her stuff in a sack and was swinging it at people. Remember that? It just broke my heart. It was very hard to take. I'm not ever going to one of those."

"I hope not." Bev says.

John leaves her alone with their visitor.

How is she coping? When did reality hit her that something was wrong?

She can't remember and admits she was in denial. She never guessed it could be something like Alzheimer's after dealing with his other health issues through the years. John has a computer, and he does fine while someone is there, but he can't do it on his own. They tackle word puzzles in the morning, and he works hard on them.

Some days he can't remember if he showered. She checks his washcloth for verification. He loves going out, but he can't remember if they went somewhere else earlier in the day.

"He forgets where things go all the time, all the time." She pauses. "I don't get to go out as much as I used to. He can't drive alone. If I do want to go shopping, he wants to go. I never get to go anywhere alone except Monday and Wednesday mornings when I go swimming. I never know what he's going to do here. I try to give him ideas. I write notes, but that doesn't do any good because he forgets to look at the notes. He's done fine so far."

Friends have come by to take him out, but not much anymore.

"He'll give them the same stories all the time. It embarrasses me sometimes because I've heard them." He asks questions and then asks them again five minutes later. "He's paying attention, but he's just not retaining anything."

It frustrates her. Their friends understand, yet have difficulties of their own. After they returned from a visitation, a friend called and said, "John looked a little lost." He has trouble interacting with a group because of the noise. He's better in a small setting.

Their family has been supportive. "They look out for us. They tease him, and he accepts it with a smile.

"I just (take care of things). I have to do it. It's a little stressful at times. I don't know if he'll get worse or not. They really don't know. We've got a lot to learn about it yet."

What frustrates me

_____

_____

_____

_____

_____

_____

Caregivers say...

Some people can't imagine being called a caregiver when caring for a loved one ... it's an unexpected job and title. Some consider it an honor and obvious responsibility. Others struggle with tending to the needs of someone who requires around-the-clock attention. Some people are natural caregivers and assume the role easily while others know themselves well enough to seek assistance. You've got to be honest with yourself. It's not just about you.

If you were or are a primary caregiver, how did you change your lifestyle or daily schedule to care for this person?

- Visited daily
- Took a second-shift job to be home during the day
- Gave up social life
- Took medical leave of absence from work
- Moved to be closer to children for assistance
- Had to retire early
- Had to move to a different house
- Had to close business
- Had to become full-time nurse, therapist and dietitian
- Gave up career to be at home
- Had to do all the driving
- Had to hire home cleaning and lawn care service
- Had to give up most of outside activities
- Had to watch him much closer
- Had to take over all the financial matters
- Called her more often
- Moved mother next door to caregiver
- Only had time for necessary shopping
- Had to get a new job to pay the bills

"We tried not to change much. We just take our time. We get a sitter if we go out together." John, 67, mother-in-law, Alzheimer's

146

▸ We hired sitters first at home during days, then 24 hours and then a nursing home. *Sylvia, 58, mother, Alzheimer's, died 17 years after diagnosed*

▸ Grandma couldn't be alone, so everyone's life pretty much had to change to adapt to her schedule. *Shallen, 25, grandmother, Alzheimer's*

▸ Making sure she was taken care of, bathing, dressing and eating right. *Jolene, 66, mother, dementia, died 5 years after diagnosed*

▸ I am not a primary, but we started to take Mom out more often to give Dad a break. *Cathi, 58, mother, dementia*

▸ We moved my folks to our town. I took a part-time job that didn't have travel. I stopped by weekly at first, then more regularly. *Ann, 49, mother, vascular dementia, died; father, Alzheimer's, died*

▸ I wake and get her medicines first thing. I take care of her all day, I'm there for PM meds, and then I'm off to bed to start all over. *Jenny, 56, mother, Alzheimer's*

▸ I gave up going to church and made him my top priority. We did what he wanted to do. *Leora, 72, husband, Alzheimer's*

▸ I drove at least once a week to care for my mother. I had to bathe her. I took her bedding and clothes home to launder. I took food. *Norma, 81, mother, Alzheimer's, died 11 years after diagnosed; sister, Alzheimer's, died 6 years after diagnosed*

▸ I quit my job to care for my father and my 93-year-old grandmother so they can stay at home. *Nettie, 51, father, Alzheimer's*

▸ She couldn't drive anymore so I took her to the hairdresser, etc., since I'm retired. *Robert, 77, wife, Alzheimer's*

▸ I took him for a lot of car rides. I didn't see much of former friends. *Edna, 83, husband, Alzheimer's, died 7 years after diagnosed*

"I do all the driving and he goes everywhere with me. He's insecure when I'm not around. He does better if he stays in familiar areas." Pat, 66, husband, Alzheimer's

▶ I did all the housework, errands during the four hours he was at day care. We had no social life and toward the end hardly left the house. He seemed afraid. *Roseann, 72, husband, dementia, died 10 years after diagnosed*

▶ So far I have a cell phone and when I leave the house, I write down in detail where I'm going and when I'll be back. *Maxine, 77, husband, Alzheimer's*

▶ Oh, yes! Your time was hers, not much for yourself. *Robert, 79, wife, Alzheimer's, died 6 years after diagnosed*

▶ I haven't let her out of my sight. *David, 69, wife, Alzheimer's*

▶ He came to live with us. I had no social life or vacation time, except when my sister visited twice a year. *Marcy, 76, father, Alzheimer's, died 5 years after diagnosed*

▶ I gave up everything to take care of him. *Shirley, 72, husband, dementia*

▶ I switched to a part-time job and assisted her with grocery shopping and paying all bills. In the six months before she moved into the long-term care center, I set out meds daily. *Judith, 61, mother, Alzheimer's*

▶ I gave up substitute teaching and church. He went with me everywhere I went. *Helen, 72, husband, Alzheimer's*

▶ I changed my business hours to by appointment. My morning schedule was changed. It was usually 10 or 11 by the time I got her fed and dressed. *Darlene, 58, mother, Alzheimer's*

▶ For a long period of time, we did everything together. Eventually I hired companions. I have had to give up putting myself first in almost any situation. *Marlene, 68, husband, dementia/Alzheimer's*

▶ My mom did the majority of the caregiving. We also had someone come during the day while my mom worked until my dad was placed in the full-care facility. *Andrew, 25, father, frontal lobe dementia, diagnosed at age 51*

▶ I didn't, except to visit her and see that she has everything she needs. I decided early on my first responsibility was to my husband, and I could not take on Mother's care at my home. I was not physically or emotionally equipped to do that. *Nancy, 65, mother, Alzheimer's*

▶ Many, many changes were necessary. We needed to bring her into our home and then ultimately into a local Alzheimer's unit. *Elizabeth, 47, mother, Alzheimer's*

▶ I quit a 20-plus year job to be with her daily while living in our home and the unit at the nursing home. *Gayle, 59, mother, Alzheimer's, died 5 years after diagnosed*

▶ I helped Mom (primary caregiver) mostly by taking care of some of the things Dad used to do (physical help). I talk and listen daily. *Mary, 38, father, Alzheimer's*

▶ I took him to work with me for two semesters, and he became our official paper shredder; then I retired early and moved to be near our children. *Sandy, 61, husband, Alzheimer's and vascular dementia*

▶ My sister and I checked in on Mom daily until she started accusing us of taking things or moving her things to try to make her think she was going crazy. *Jody, 47, mother, early onset Alzheimer's*

▶ All of my free time for a long time was dedicated to getting her things in order. It turned out she was swindled by a number of people, and I had to go to battle with these people. It was very painful. *Kevin, 45, mother, Alzheimer's*

149

What changes have I made?

_____

_____

_____

_____

_____

_____

"I don't see Dad as a guy with Alzheimer's"

Megan and Brad are two siblings who have had to grow up far too fast and learn the true meaning of sacrifice. They've devoted a huge portion of their teen and young adult years to caring for their father who has Alzheimer's.

The brother and sister faced some difficult challenges and traumatic experiences in their teens, including the loss of their mother to cancer. Six months later, their dad was also diagnosed with cancer. Megan remembers: "We were so nervous about losing him that we took him up to Mayo Clinic every six months." It was then they learned he also had Alzheimer's.

"He was an accountant," she says. "His co-workers informed us. You notice it pretty quickly when you're in a job where you have to be so exact." His associates bought the business from him when Megan was in college. "They still let him work part time and checked over what he did. I think our mom covered up for him a lot. Socially, she was a huge talker, so you wouldn't notice him repeating himself. He finally got his chance to talk when she passed away." She laughs at the sad irony.

How did they decide to take on this full-time role?

"We didn't really sit down and talk about it," Megan says. "We just never saw it any other way. He's our dad. We're going to take care of him."

"He would do the same thing for us," Brad says. He lost his mom to cancer when he was only 15. One day, he and his girlfriend were cleaning house, and they found some letters from his dad to his mom when he was in the military. "He used to be like me. I could easily be like this some day. How would I like to be treated? It was neat seeing how he talked and acted. I don't see him as a guy with Alzheimer's. He is a human being."

Brad was 16 and still in high school when his dad started taking one drug. In the beginning, his dad didn't need as much assistance, but when Brad reached college, he realized he had to do more. He'd go home instead of out with friends, and he says he's missed a lot of "ordinary" everyday life while caring for his dad. He's put his career on hold, but fortunately his employer has been supportive by allowing him to work irregular hours.

They had considered other options in the beginning when both siblings were working days, Brad says. A girl they knew came over during the day to check on their dad and made sure he ate, but he didn't take to that at all. They're not sure why, but it could have been that in his mind he didn't need the help. It made it him mad. He wandered off in a huff, and they couldn't let him do that. Brad decided to stay home during the day.

When ask if he feels resentful, he says he doesn't, though admits it can be frustrating. His friends probably have no idea what it's like for him. An out-of-town relative calls to tell all that she's doing.

" 'That's nice,' " he says. " 'We were home with Dad all weekend.' It's like they don't get it sometimes."

Megan adds, "I remember being on spring break in college and not having as much fun as I should, worrying about things back home. I've learned so much. I know about so many things other people don't. It definitely balanced out. I've had to give up going out on weekends, but that's okay.

"I know I'm doing the right thing. People tell us a lot, 'We really respect you for what you're doing.' " This teacher met her husband at a speed dating event and laughs, "It was all I had time for. He's been totally understanding and helps Dad all the time. All my friends are having babies right now. We're in no hurry. I feel horrible for Brad, who hasn't been able to get a full-time job yet. But I know good things will happen to him for all he has done."

Both attended a variety of workshops at the local Alzheimer's Association and praised the assistance and guidance they gathered as they prepared for the caregiver experience.

"I took the sessions because I don't like surprises," Megan says. "I wanted to know. I know the next thing will be changes going to the bathroom." She's already studied what kind of clothes might work best. "I try to stay prepared for everything so I can handle it when it does comes. I wasn't prepared when my mom died, and that was the hardest part of it. I don't want to feel that way again. (For 10 years) Mom always beat it, so we figured she would beat it again. We weren't expecting her to … She had been getting better and all of a sudden, she passed away."

Brad says they've witnessed their father going back further in his memories. He can't remember what he did today, but he can recall the first and last names of classmates. He still remembers them, but he has days when he asks, "Where's Brad?" Sometimes their dad asks, "Where's Mom?" They're not sure if he's asking about his wife or his own mother.

In everyday care, he says they only make him shower every two or three days because he won't do it on his own now. "We don't like to push him to do anything he doesn't want to do. He gets frustrated. It's often a challenge as it takes a while. Pick your battles. It's hard to remember what it was like back a few years ago since he's gotten worse. Megan and I take care of him ... like parents. It's flipped."

His sister concurs with that role reversal.

"I'm trying to make changes as comfortable as possible for him," Megan explains. He's going to require more help in bathing, and she's been giving him manicures and pedicures to help him adjust to her touching him. She washes his hair in the sink. "We're not a real touchy, huggy family, so I'm easing him into that. We're trying to stay a step ahead of him."

At the same time, they don't smother him. Brad believes their dad thinks he's alone and doesn't realize they're there with him, which probably gives him a sense of independence. His dad will ask him why he's home, and Brad just tells him he's got the day off. That answer satisfies him.

"We're trying to be as sensitive as possible," Megan says, "so that he still thinks he's doing more of it. He helps me carry things out to the car, fold clothes, get me a glass of milk. I know that sounds really lazy, but I know he can still do that, and he likes doing things for me. Little things like that."

It does no good to give him things that will frustrate him. Her teaching experience also helps as she gives him ways to communicate by answering questions and keeps his mind working. "He loves to talk. He's still amazing at spelling. He's a walking dictionary. He loves to run errands with me, being in the car and pushing the grocery cart. It was weird, I went to the grocery store the other night by myself. You mean I have to push the cart?" She laughs.

When she's in a bad mood, he's in a bad mood. "He's not sure why. But if I'm in a great mood, he's in that mood." So she has to watch her moods carefully. "If he takes a nap and wakes up, he's usually in a good mood." She's learned some valuable advice as a first grade teacher. What she's applied in the classroom has helped her be a better and more patient caregiver.

"They're similar in so many ways."

How do people respond to their father in public situations?

He's still an intelligent man, Megan says, and it's upsetting when people talk down to him. She admits that they do kind of shelter him. He's not wanted to go to church anymore because their church has become crowded, and they decided to go to a smaller congregation. He's uncomfortable running into people he doesn't remember. At the grocery store he sometimes knows someone. "Sometimes he doesn't, and I don't either, but they know him, and we just laugh about it."

B rad says some neighbors have stopped by, taken their dad out to lunch or someplace else. "Things like that have been really nice. Just treat him like the same person he always was. It's nice when people ask my Dad, 'How are you? Haven't seen you in a while.' Rather than them asking us 'How's your dad?' we'd rather you talk to him and treat him like he's still there. Send a card or something. It's not like we're trying to get someone to volunteer to take care of him.

"We noticed how differently people treated my dad when they knew he had Alzheimer's. He's still the same person. It's not like he has no idea what's going on around him."

A relative overheard someone one day making fun of their father, how it was his fault he had the disease, how he made mistakes. That's very painful, Brad says.

"What's hurtful is how people don't call him anymore. We have family we used to be with once a month, and they probably haven't called in years. One said they didn't call because they didn't know if he'd answer, but he still knows who they are. Even if he doesn't answer, they can leave a message. They just don't get it, I guess. But I'm not saying I wouldn't be the same way."

Megan says, "People will ask, 'How's your dad?' I'll say fine because they don't really want to hear it."

How do they keep each other motivated?

"It's nice to have someone else," Brad says. "If I was doing it alone, it would be stressful and depressing. We're lucky." His wife and Megan's husband have been tremendous help. He says he's not one to let things bother him. When people ask if he's okay, he reassures them he is. He's looking forward to the future. From what he's witnessed, other families have it much worse than what they've experienced.

"Every minute of our day is planned around him. He has the disease, but it affects every single hour of our lives. Everything else is secondary. My dad comes first. It affects the caregiver more than the person with the disease. I'm glad to help, but it's like a thankless job because the person you're helping out doesn't realize it. I can't work full-time, I don't get benefits, I don't get anything from the government for taking care of my dad. That doesn't seem right in a way."

What's his advice to families faced with a similar situation? Educate yourself. Some things are hard to face and may make you want to "run away," he says. People will tell you things, but you still have to face it yourself. People could read all about it, but they actually have to go through it to fully comprehend it.

Megan reads of many other caregivers burning out. She stresses that they must "always make time for themselves. Everything I read on boards about people who have no other time. You can't do everything yourself. That's the hardest part. You have to realize that you don't have to do everything. We want to keep him at home as long as possible. He's happy, he's comfortable, and that's why he's done so well because there's been no major changes."

Are there things their dad has said and done that have surprised or amused Megan?

"Every day." Megan laughs. People assume it's a huge chore or wonder how they do it. "But he's so happy that we're here with him, and he's so appreciative of what we do for him. When I cook for him, he'll say, 'Megan, that's so delicious.' And half the time, it's not. He's just so nice. He's always making jokes about things. It's not hard. I know it will get hard. When it does get harder, we'll remember how appreciative he's been for so long. That will make things so much easier."

Caregivers say...

Each of us has priorities and defines sacrifices differently. Something of importance to one person is insignificant to another, and that's hard for some onlookers to understand. Caregivers should not be ashamed of lamenting these losses.

What were some of the personal items or events that you had to give up to be a caregiver?

▶ Almost everything

▶ Time

▶ Had to arrange new work schedule

▶ Taking vacations

▶ Ability to leave home anytime I wanted

▶ Less contact with family and friends

▶ Financial freedom

▶ Church and choir

▶ Group social activities

▶ Holidays

▶ Hobbies

▶ Profession

▶ Piano lessons

▶ Dining out with friends

▶ Entertaining at home

▶ Personal freedom

▶ Time away together, but we still get time. It's very important. *John, 67, mother-in-law, Alzheimer's*

▶ Nothing. We included Mom and her caregiver in everything. *Jolene, 66, mother, dementia, died 5 years after diagnosed*

▶ We just shifted responsibilities and locations of holidays. *Cathi, 58, mother, dementia*

▶ Freedom, going places without him. I'd like to take art classes, but we're about to the point where I could do more things and just take him. *June, 66, husband, early onset Alzheimer's*

▶ Time. Everything revolved around her needs and care. *Gayle, 59, mother, Alzheimer's, died 5 years after diagnosed*

▶ My two teen-agers and husband were very supportive. I did miss some things like sewing for my daughter. *Norma, 81, mother, Alzheimer's, died 11 years after diagnosed; sister, Alzheimer's, died 6 years after diagnosed*

156

- I had to give up having weekends to unwind at the end of the work week. *Mary Ann, 62, father, Alzheimer's*

- My own home and getting paid. *Nettie, 51, father, Alzheimer's*

- I couldn't fish and hunt as much. *Robert, 77, wife, Alzheimer's*

- It was difficult to be gone for more than two-three days during this last year. I checked on her one to two times a day. *Judith, 61, mother, Alzheimer's*

- I guess I had to give up helping others, tinkering with my tools, our dancing. *Robert, 79, wife, Alzheimer's, died 6 years after diagnosed*

- Trips, sit-down time, peace of mind. I was always worried. *Marcy, 76, father, Alzheimer's, died 5 years after diagnosed*

- All of my wants/needs have become unimportant. *Marlene, 68, husband, dementia/Alzheimer's*

- We couldn't travel much. It was difficult to attend social gatherings. Because of us losing so much money, I didn't buy much for myself. I also quit taking two prescriptions. *Vicky, 54, husband, early onset Alzheimer's, died 5 years after diagnosed*

- Myself. No time for that. *Marcy, 76, husband, memory loss due to massive stroke*

- I was still in college during his initial diagnosis and realized I needed to return home after college to help. *Andrew, 25, father, frontal lobe dementia, diagnosed at age 51*

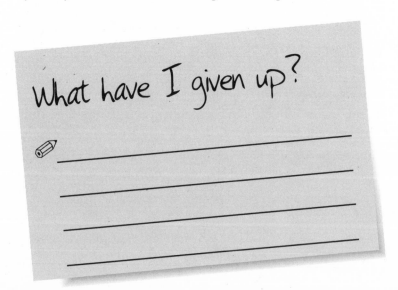

What have I given up?

Caregivers say...

Everyone responds differently to making sacrifices. That's part of who we are as human beings.

How did you feel about what you had to give up?   157

- Frustrated
- Sad
- No reluctance
- Sorry for him
- Didn't mind
- Overwhelmed
- Tired
- Resentful

- Angry
- Emotionally and physically drained
- Isolated at first
- Alone
- Okay
- Compensated in other ways

- My whole life, goals and dreams are now completely changed. Sometimes I feel angry, but it was the right thing to do. It is just a very different life. *Christl, 55, father, stroke and Alzheimer's*

- My mom was always strong and took care of herself, home and a large garden. Seeing her change made me sad and troubled. *Jolene, 66, mother, dementia, died 5 years after diagnosed*

- Torn, but decisive. I wouldn't have had it otherwise. I do think it negatively impacted my parenting to my son. He had ADD and got into legal trouble about the same time. He started drinking alcohol in eighth grade. As a reaction for attention? *Ann, 49, mother, vascular dementia, died; father, Alzheimer's, died*

Caregiving is okay if ...ewed positively." *John, 67, ...other-in-law, Alzheimer's*

- Sad, but glad to still be together. It created more work for us, but it is important. *Cathi, 58, mother, dementia*

▸ I try not to think about it and just make do with what we do still have together. Many times though I feel very alone. *Pat, 66, husband, Alzheimer's*

▸ Sometimes it makes me angry, then I feel guilty, then I feel sad. But I want to give her a few good years. We do a lot together. *Jenny, 56, mother, Alz-heimer's*

158

▸ I didn't like it but accepted it, knowing it would change some day. *Leora, 72, husband, Alzheimer's*

▸ Somewhat stressed, juggling my own world and Dad's needs, but very willing to do it for Dad. *Mary Ann, 62, father, Alzheimer's*

▸ I was tired. I had to give up some of my hobbies and being gone one day a week. I had to get my home, etc., in order in less time. *Norma, 81, mother, Alzheimer's, died 11 years after diagnosed; sister, Alzheimer's, died 6 years after diagnosed*

▸ Good, blessed. I grew up with great parents and grandparents, and this is the least I can do. *Nettie, 51, father, Alzheimer's*

▸ She said we were "not married anymore." That hurt a lot. *Robert, 77, wife, Alzheimer's*

▸ It had to be done. *Phil, 69, mother, dementia*

▸ Because of the dementia, I felt bad because of the things we as a couple couldn't do, places we couldn't go. *Roseann, 72, husband, dementia, died 10 years after diagnosed*

▸ If he can't or won't go, I wouldn't be interested in going, so I feel okay. *Maxine, 77, husband, Alzheimer's*

▸ I really did not think of how I felt. My concern was for her. I was going to try to be there for her as long as my health would let me. *Robert, 79, wife, Alzheimer's, died 6 years after diagnosed*

▸ Glad that I could make her life as pleasant as possible. *Ann, 63, aunt, Alzheimer's, died 6 years after diagnosed*

▸ In a way "lost." *David, 69, wife, Alzheimer's*

"Slightly depressed. It put stress on my marriage." Darlene, 58, mother, Alzheimer's

▸ By end of five years, my stomach was in knots. I was afraid I would be in no condition to live a normal life again. *Marcy, 76, father, Alzheimer's, died 5 years after diagnosed*

▸ She needed me and appreciated what I did. We became closer than ever. *Judith, 61, mother, Alzheimer's*

▸ Sad, angry, powerful, unappreciated. I go through periods of being angry at him. Sometimes it feels like I'm pulling up old issues, and I find myself saying under my breath, "Well, you always were selfish and nothing has changed." I can't hang on to past hurts and deal with now at the same time. *Marlene, 68, husband, dementia/Alzheimer's*

▸ Sad that she was missing those events as well. *Kim, 34, grandmother, died 5 years after diagnosed*

▸ It was an honor. I would do it again in a flash. *Gayle, 59, mother, Alzheimer's, died 5 years after diagnosed*

▸ I felt very cheated and lonely. Lonely because I didn't feel I could confide in anyone about the money issues. *Vicky, 54, husband, early onset Alzheimer's, died 5 years after diagnosed*

▸ Tired. My resentment lessened over time. *Marcy, 76, husband, memory loss due to massive stroke*

▸ It gave me a sense of purpose. I felt an obligation to my family to help in any way possible. *Andrew, 25, father, frontal lobe dementia, diagnosed at age 51*

▸ Okay most of the time. It wears on you after a while. *Chris, 51, mother, Alzheimer's*

▸ Sad and worried that I am not taking care of my health problems. *Martha, 71, husband, cognitive decline*

▸ It wasn't easy. *Bill, 78, wife, Alzheimer's, died 4 years after diagnosed*

▸ I was happy to care for my mother. I was saddened by watching her lose more and more of herself. *Sally, 57, mother, Alzheimer's, died 3 years after diagnosed*

"In many ways just matter-of-fact. That's what families do." Mary, 38, father, Alzheimer's

Just talking...

(Caregiver and client responses and reactions are in italics.)

At the opening of the latest round of support group sessions for recently diagnosed clients and their immediate caregivers, veterans and newcomers introduce themselves in the circle.

A wife makes everyone chuckle as she tells of looking for her husband one day. Finally she found him disassembling the water hose attachment to the house. His response to her dismay? "Why it is you always show up when I don't want you to?" Her answer? "Because you're a very lucky man."

A usually quiet male client points to his wife and announces to everyone's chagrin, "I don't know which one of us belongs here ..."

Bonnie, a facilitator, explains that memory loss is like an electrical short in the brain. The nerve paths can't transmit information properly. You can't tell someone to concentrate harder to make it better. There are good and bad times every day.

"Why can you forget something today and remember it three days later?"

"I don't know," she admits.

"Okay." Everyone laughs.

"Prayers and songs stay with you," one spouse says.

Bonnie says researchers don't understand why some memories stay and others vanish, but it all depends on what portion of the brain is affected. Music and sensitivity to certain emotions seem to remain longer. They often find that music makes clients responsive when they've not spoken in a long time.

As the caregivers gather with Bonnie, she reminds them that their loved one probably doesn't want to be pigeonholed by being labeled in one stage or another of dementia because there is no exact science to predicting what symptoms of what stage will present themselves at any time.

"We have to plan for tomorrow, but what are their abilities today?" She looks around the room. "The caregivers are adapting. The clients are *not* adapting."

The disease itself often makes them unaware of their condition. Bonnie says she lied to her mother when she told her she didn't have dementia. Her mother then said she was luckier than the other people at the assisted living facility because "I don't have what they have."

A wife says her husband now tells people he has Alzheimer's. He doesn't ask to drive, gets frustrated when he can't do something and is sleeping more. His afternoons are now the best time of the day.

Bonnie says some medications can affect how their day goes and there may be better times to take them. She suggests all of them keep notes on how their loved one responds to medication so they can share that with the doctor, as that may affect the type, dosage and time it's administered.

161

A spouse says her husband now has trouble identifying the door.

Memory loss affects depth perception and vision. For example, a client may not be able to see the salt at the end of the table because their placemat may be their whole world at that moment.

One client is now putting garbage in the refrigerator.

Several indicate that their loved ones are sleeping more.

"Our folks sleep a lot," Bonnie says. "It bothers us, but it doesn't bother them."

A wife tells everyone how her husband has now been diagnosed with cancer and is going downhill. He won't drink and is dehydrated. His doctor suggested she give him two small breath mints and pretend they're medicine to get him to drink. Tell him it's a cocktail when she gives him cranberry juice at night.

"He's tired of hearing my voice."

Individuals with Alzheimer's lose their appetite and grasp on reality. Bonnie says caregivers must decide what is really important and make everything as simple as they can.

Another reports that her loved one is the fifth member of the family to be diagnosed with Alzheimer's.

A wife explains that she had suspected for a long time that something was not right with her husband. He's had an anger problem with not being allowed to drive. New medications have helped in calming him. "He's sleeping more. I'm glad to hear from all of you that others are, too. I thought I was going to lose my mind for several months."

"We must remember the quality of life and safety," Bonnie says. "It's a hard decision to keep them safe, but it is a disease."

Some clients experience paranoia. Women are often easy targets because some males with dementia accuse their wives of fooling around with other men after they've been to the beauty salon as always. At moments like that, it's hard to accept this as a disease. That's why "we can't lose our sense of humor."

A daughter reports that her mother, who has Alzheimer's, is lashing out at her father. She's getting mean and loud.

"Sadly, I lost my temper," she says as her tears flow.

"Congratulations," Bonnie says gently, "you're human."

Everyone reassures her that it's okay to cry.

One woman says her family doesn't believe anything's wrong with her husband. They doubt her while "he's been on a stage performing."

"Our bathroom is redecorated every day. It's like a hunt," a spouse says with a smile.

The group is quite lively one afternoon as Bonnie and Jenn try to get them to settle down for a productive session. It's more like a class of kids eager for spring break.

"How is everybody?" Jenn asks.

"Hunky dory!" says one.

"I don't remember," announces another, drawing a chorus of laughs.

Smiling, Bonnie shakes her head. "I can tell how this evening is going to go. How was your Easter with all your family?"

"All the freeloaders."

Yes, it's going to be one of those days ...

How do I really feel?

Discovering & rediscovering the beauty of everyday life

"Just because the people with Alzheimer's have lost their memories, that doesn't mean that you lose those memories, too. You should cherish every minute."
Shallen, 25, grandmother, Alzheimer's

No more excuses!

Here's what you can say & do

So, you claim you don't know what to say to or do for individuals with dementia or memory loss and their immediate caregivers? There are suggestions scattered throughout this entire volume, but with this section, you have no more excuses! The use of the word "them" can be either the person with dementia or the caregiver or both, whatever best suits your situation.

▶ *Bring magazines featuring photos or short bits of information on a favorite hobby or sport.*

▶ *Bring books or magazines featuring colorful photos of nature and scenes from around the world or favorite locations.*

▶ *Bring library books.*

▶ *Bring books on audio.*

▶ *Record your voice telling a favorite story or memory.*

▶ *Offer to read aloud.*

▶ *Find some audio CDs with sound effects and create a game out of guessing the sounds.*

▶ *Find articles or books that include memories written by people the same age.*

▶ *Find CDs of music from the era in which they grew up.*

▶ *Find audio recordings of famous speeches.*

▶ *Do you play a musical instrument? Make the sound level enjoyable enough for a personal concert.*

▶ *Do you sing? Give them a personal concert.*

▶ *Do you love to act? Give them a personal show.*

▶ *Offer to take them to the library, the park, public gardens, the zoo, a petting farm, a museum or a historical home.*

▶ *Offer to take them to watch a high school football game or a baseball game in the park or children on the playground.*

▶ *Offer to take them on a drive through the country and look for grazing animals and old barns.*

▶ *Offer to take them on a picnic with a real basket and blanket.*

▶ *Offer to take them to a band concert in the park or at a special event.*

▶ *Offer to take them to festivals only if they are not bothered by crowds, or pick the least crowded time to attend, or just walk around the perimeter to pick up sights, sounds and aromas without being overwhelmed.*

▶ *Offer to take them to the county or 4-H fair. Buy them a lemonade shake-up or elephant ear (if it's okay for their diet).*

▶ *Offer to take them to pick apples in an orchard, pumpkins or strawberries in the field.*

▶ *Offer to take them to the farmers' market or to plant sales.*

▶ *Bring basic art supplies such as crayons, watercolor paints or drawing pads.*

▶ *Bring some packs of stickers and create funny pictures.*

▶ *Look through old catalogues or collectors' books of products to spark memories of household items, clothes, old toys, dishware, appliances, sports equipment.*

▶ *Buy some interesting scrapbook pages that feature topics of interest.*

▶ *Offer to take care of non-personal laundry like sheets and towels.*

▶ *Run errands at a regular time every week, two weeks, etc.*

Just use your common sense!

One caregiver suggests a reverse gift list. Think of what you do in your everyday life, and that's what the caregiver needs done. If you've got trash, they've got trash. If you've got a water softener that needs salt, they likely have one, too.

If you eat, there's a good chance they do, too.

"It's easy for me to put on paper, but it's not always easy for someone else to execute. I'd sometimes leave a 'to do list' on the counter, hoping the kids would see it. More often, they found it easier to buy me a plant. Just give me one whole Saturday …"

More often than not, a caregiver won't ask for help. That's why others need to come up with a "here's how I can help you" list.

Digging not-so-deep to find out more about your loved one

You can get to know more about your loved one in many ways:

▶ *Talk to neighbors or friends or distant relatives who may offer unique insight or memories.*

▶ *Talk to fellow members of organizations that they belonged to through the years, including religious and social groups.*

▶ *Look at their old photos.*

▶ *Go through old high school and college yearbooks.*

▶ *Find letters they had written years before.*

▶ *Look at the types of movies, music or books they collect.*

▶ *Find out what kind of work and/or hobbies this person has been involved with over the years.*

▶ *Have grandchildren ask about games they used to play as a child.*

Involve the whole family

If you have some relatives who have distanced themselves during the caregiving process, invite them to contribute memories, copies of old home movies, photos, letters, etc. That's a non-threatening way for them to be involved. If you break some barriers by doing this, you may be able to dismantle more walls along the way.

No what matter what anybody contributes, let them know that their contribution has made a difference. For example, show them a photo of your loved one enjoying looking at old photos or home movies. Make an audio or video recording of memories that they may share while looking at these.

Share with them photos of your loved one playing with pets or children, being creative, walking in the park ... and stopping to smell the roses.

Making those memories

Make memory boxes to help loved ones recall favorite hobbies, objects, people and events in their lives. They can be a collection of items or themed to spark memories. Involve them in the process of creating them. Here are an abundance of topics:

167

▶ Spouse	▶ Drama, comedy
▶ Children	▶ Toys, stuffed animals
▶ Grandchildren	▶ Stamps, coins
▶ Parents	▶ Collectibles
▶ Grandparents	▶ Weather
▶ Siblings	▶ Hunting, fishing
▶ School	▶ Nature
▶ Religious	▶ Ocean
▶ Tools	▶ Vacations
▶ Home maintenance	▶ Around the world
▶ Woodworking	▶ Heritage
▶ Kitchen	▶ Hometown
▶ Nursery	▶ Friends
▶ Sewing	▶ Neighborhood
▶ Knitting, crocheting	▶ Awards
▶ Gardening	▶ Recipes, favorite foods
▶ Cooking	▶ Career, profession
▶ Auto repair	▶ Previous homes
▶ Auto sports	▶ _____
▶ Team sports	▶ _____
▶ Individual sports	▶ _____
▶ Books	▶ _____
▶ Photography	▶ _____
▶ Music	▶ _____
▶ Art	

History 101

Revisiting important events in history may stir a conversation about where they were when headlines were made. Of course, it all depends on the era and location in which they grew up. For example, events in United States history:

Witnessing history

▸ *The Great Depression*

▸ *Start of World War II*

▸ *The draft*

▸ *Relatives in the service*

▸ *Rationing on the homefront*

▸ *Victory gardens*

▸ *Franklin D. Roosevelt's death*

▸ *End of World War II*

▸ *Harry S. Truman*

▸ *Korea*

▸ *The Cold War*

▸ *Bomb shelters*

▸ *The Edsel*

▸ *Dwight D. Eisenhower*

▸ *Sputnik*

▸ *First Americans in space*

▸ *John F. Kennedy*

▸ *Cuban missile crisis*

▸ *Civil Rights movement*

▸ *Kennedy's assassination*

▸ *Vietnam War*

▸ *Lyndon B. Johnson*

▸ *Martin Luther King Jr.*

▸ *Woodstock, the hippie era*

▸ *Politics*

▸ *Richard M. Nixon*

▸ *Watergate*

▸ *Gas shortages*

Entertainment & social history

▸ *Radio shows*

▸ *Movie matinees*

▸ *Saturday night*

▸ *Television*

▸ *Movie stars*

▸ *Hit records*

▸ *Automobiles*

▸ *Baseball*

▸ *Football*

▸ *Olympics*

▸ *World's Fairs*

▸ *Hobbies*

▸ *Going on vacation*

▸ *Fads*

Stirring up memories of long, long ago

Many individuals with Alzheimer's tend to go back in time, remembering long-term events better than short-term. When your loved one is in the mood to reminisce, consider some of these topics to encourage memories. And be sure to record them!

The earliest memories of ...

- *Childhood*
- *Mother*
- *Father*
- *Brothers and sisters*
- *Grandparents*
- *Great-grandparents*
- *Aunts and uncles*
- *Cousins*
- *Home*
- *School*
- *Teachers*
- *Friends*

- *Enemies*
- *Religious events*
- *Role models*
- *Jobs*
- *Family vacations*
- *Falling in love*
- *Married life*
- *Having children*
- _____
- _____
- _____
- _____

The first ...

- *Day of school*
- *Love*
- *Date*
- *Kiss*
- *Automobile*
- *Job*

- _____
- _____
- _____
- _____
- _____
- _____

The to-do and can-do file: Rediscover their history

When the weather's nice, or at least tolerable during the hottest and coldest months, turn an excursion outside into an uplifting adventure for a loved one with dementia or memory loss. It can be a joyous rediscovery of life's simplest things for both of you.

Determine the physical capabilities, interest and attention span of your loved one to find out how far they can go for how long. And remember to take a tape recorder or video camera — as long as it doesn't distract them or make them uncomfortable. You will discover some priceless memories and stories you've never heard before.

If they are physically unable to leave their home or health-care facility, use personal photos, historical books about their community, school yearbooks, textures and scents to make for an enjoyable journey for both of you.

A walk around the yard

When was the last time you took a stroll around your own back yard? Walk every corner and take a closer look at each of the bushes, trees and flowers. Go several times during all seasons for different sensations.

▶ *What colors and flowers do they like?*

▶ *What scents grab their attention?*

▶ *What textures do they like?*

▶ *Is there a special history or story about any of the plants or trees?*

▶ *Were they involved in the planting or care for some or all?*

▶ *Are there stumps of trees the kids used to climb?*

▶ *Did they plant seedlings from a school science project?*

▶ *Was there a rose bush that supplied fresh roses for the dinner table?*

▶ *What were the pains of mowing the yard and types of equipment?*

▶ *Were there plants or trees that one person loved and another hated?*

▶ *Where was the kids' swing set? Who used to fall off the slide? Who would swing for hours?*

▶ *Where was the sandbox? Where was the kiddie pool?*

▶ *Was there a bird feeder? What kind of birds appeared? How did they keep the squirrels out of the feeder? Was there a bird bath?*

▶ *Was there a vegetable garden? What was served fresh for meals?*

▶ *What kind of colors do they remember?*

▶ *What were the pleasant scents and bad odors?*

▶ *Did they used to have cookouts in the back yard? Who attended? What was served? What did everybody wear?*

▶ *What holidays were celebrated there? What was the Fourth of July like with all the sparklers?*

|7|

A walk through the neighborhood

Have they lived here all their life or for decades? Start a conversation about who used to live in what house and how the street has changed. You'll discover something new every time depending on the direction you walk, the weather, and time of day or year. See if a neighbor will allow you to explore their yard, vegetable or flower gardens to stimulate the senses with different scents and textures. Ask some of the same questions as noted previously.

A walk through the childhood neighborhood

If it's a convenient drive, visit the neighborhood and house where your loved one grew up. Use some of the questions suggested previously and add these:

▶ *Where was their bedroom? Who did they have to share it with?*

▶ *How was it decorated? Where did they store their toys and games? What were their favorite belongings and clothes? Did the closet or under the bed used to scare them? Did they used to read by flashlight under the blankets?*

▶ *What was the layout of the house? What was the most popular room? What was their favorite piece of furniture? Did Dad and Mom have favorite chairs? What were they doing while sitting?*

▶ *Where was the radio and television? What were the favorite shows? What night was special to gather around them?*

▸ *Where was the bathroom? Did it have an old tub? How many people shared that bathroom? Did they have to wait in line?*

▸ *Where was the kitchen? What did it smell and look like? What were some of their favorite and least favorite meals? Did they used to slip food to the dog? Was everybody home for dinner every night?*

▸ *Who were the kids they grew up with? What were their favorite games? Where was the neighborhood hangout? Clubhouse? Tree house?*

▸ *Did the front porch have a swing? Did it creak? Were there rocking chairs or other furniture?*

▸ *Which relatives used to visit most often? Who were they anxious to see? Who did they hide from?*

▸ *How it was decorated for the holidays, inside and out?*

▸ *What autos used to be parked in the driveways or alleys?*

▸ *Did they walk or ride the bus to school? Who did they go with?*

▸ *Who were the senior citizens down the street? Who was friendly? Who was cranky?*

A walk by the old school

Walk or drive by their old schools.

▸ *Did they walk or ride the bus to school?*

▸ *What grades did they attend there?*

▸ *Was there one entrance or separate ones for boys and girls?*

▸ *Where were their classrooms?*

▸ *Who were some of their teachers?*

▸ *Who were some of their classmates?*

▸ *What did they like or love about school?*

▸ *What did they hate about school?*

▸ *What were their favorite and least favorite subjects?*

▸ *What did they do at recess?*

▸ *Did they take their lunch or go home everyday?*

▸ *Were they in the school band, choir or theatrical group?*

▸ *Did they ever win a spelling bee, math contest, etc.?*

- *What was the first school dance they attended?*
- *Did they play sports?*
- *What was their team mascot? School colors?*
- *Do they remember the school song?*
- *Did they attend homecoming parades?*
- *Did they go to the prom?*
- *How did they feel when they graduated?*

A walk through the park

Public parks will look different during every season as flowers and trees bloom and fade. Create a fall leaf collection just like you made in school. An assortment of colors and textures will stimulate memories, as will the sound and sight of leaves being raked. Parks are generally big enough to visit a different section every day for weeks.

Encourage the use of all the senses where possible: touch, sight, sound, smell and taste. These can ignite powerful and pleasant memories.

What can we do and see?

_____

_____

_____

_____

_____

_____

_____

_____

A little creativity and patience go a long way

When it comes to engaging someone with dementia or memory loss, patient and family services coordinator Alisha has "learned to go with the flow."

While working at an assisted living facility before joining the Alzheimer's Association, she discovered that, "I might have scheduled programs or certain activities, but the residents may not feel like painting. Maybe they want to play a card game or just need some time to relax or have some soft music in the background. It was very much up to me to read each person individually and know what their needs were."

Families can do the same, she says.

For example, one woman didn't want to be around crowds because her anxiety levels would skyrocket. However, she couldn't express those feelings and fears verbally, so she "acted out." Alisha would escort her back to her room and sit quietly with her. By observation, she learned what this woman liked, could do and what level of social interaction was comfortable.

That's what she encourages families to do as they cope with a loved one's Alzheimer's or related disorder. Find out the specific needs and be as creative with that as possible.

Laughter is very important, and people can laugh about absolutely nothing because it truly is contagious. She's found that she can start to laugh for no reason, and dementia and memory loss clients will join in. That simple act can make anybody feel better emotionally and physically. Learn to make light of a situation when the individual forgets something. That eases the stress and frustration.

Music continues to be a major connection with clients. Learn what music is important to them, such as tunes from their childhood or religious hymns. These can often be played repeatedly because it brings them joy. She'd like to see more karoke programs available for older songs from the 1930s-1950s.

Incorporate music and exercise because it adds a beat and fun. Even if they're only tapping their toes, that's still positive and gets them moving.

Asking for
& accepting
assistance

"There are many adjustments in our lives to keep Mom home with us. My husband agreed to Mom coming here, but if he saw it was too much for me, he would step in and talk about other options. My concern: How long can I do this?"
Jenny, 56, mother, Alzheimer's

Caregivers say...

If you love someone, you have an emotional and physical bond with them. When they're hurting, you're hurting.

176 **How were or have you been affected emotionally and physically by all this?**

- Much more sensitive to caregivers and elders
- Gained weight
- Lost weight
- Tired and sad
- Empty
- Lamenting loss of a good friend
- More emotional
- Depressed
- Worried about the future
- Stressed
- Trouble sleeping
- Quieter, almost unsocial
- Developed high blood pressure
- It's very draining
- Anxiety attacks
- Prayed more often
- Emotional rollercoaster
- Frustration
- Exhaustion
- Back pain from lifting and bending
- Heartbroken
- Better and stronger person
- Occasionally have a good cry

- I've grown from the experience as did my entire family. *Sylvia, 58, mother, Alzheimer's, died 17 years after diagnosed*
- The staff at the nursing home is very kind to me. *Robert, 77, wife, Alzheimer's*

- I really couldn't plan anything. I went on a vacation and had to cut it short. *Jolene, 66, mother, dementia, died 5 years after diagnosed*
- I don't have time to be emotional or physical. *David, 69, wife, Alzheimer's*

"Sometimes I need to get out and breathe or clear my mind." Nettie, 51, father, Alzheimer's

▸ I had to move out of our bedroom due to nightmares he physically reacts to. It was hard to sleep alone. *Pat, 66, husband, Alzheimer's*

▸ Emotionally it's hard. Keep the stiff upper lip and all. Physically and emotionally I feel drained, tired, sad, angry, guilty, alone, scared. *Jenny, 56, mother, Alzheimer's*

▸ It seems like I've lost my spirit, my sense of humor. I'm tired. I feel and look old. *Roseann, 72, husband, dementia, died 10 years after diagnosed*

▸ Physically it took a lot of energy; emotionally it was very sad to watch my parent become the child. *Anne, 67, mother, dementia, died 4 years after diagnosed*

▸ It impacts all of my decisions … to travel, to move, expenses, family time. *Elizabeth, 47, mother, Alzheimer's*

▸ I felt maternal and protective towards her. *Kim, 34, grandmother, died 5 years after diagnosed*

▸ My husband said nicely that I had aged 10 years. It made me a better and more patient person. *Gayle, 59, mother, Alzheimer's, died 5 years after diagnosed*

▸ Emotionally it has been like an extended grieving process that you still can't complete or have closure. *Andrew, 25, father, frontal lobe dementia, diagnosed at age 51*

▸ I cry much more easily. *Martha, 71, husband, cognitive decline*

▸ "How wasn't I" is the better question. It affects everyone, even my teenager. *Mary, 38, father, Alzheimer's*

▸ Emotionally, I feel she has very little good quality of life and wish she would peacefully pass on. *J, grandmother, Alzheimer's*

▸ I call on the Lord, out loud in many situations, and He helps. Deeper faith, dearer friends. *Catherine, 85, husband, Alzheimer's and Lewy Body*

"Gradually I'm learning patience and that I can do more than I thought." *June, 66, husband, early onset Alzheimer's*

Just talking...

(Caregiver and client responses and reactions are in italics.)

Communication: it's so easy, yet so hard.

Clients and caregivers tune in as Alzheimer's Association facilitators Alisha and Bonnie remind them that communication is crucial in keeping everyone informed about the changes a loved one experiences with dementia or memory loss. High on that priority list is educating everyone on what to expect and how to cope.

A caregiver says a daughter, who lives a couple of hundred miles away, struggles to accept her father's diagnosis when he sounds fine on the telephone.

"It may be hard being far away and not seeing it every day," says Alisha.

Bonnie concurs that it's often hard to explain it to someone who's not witnessing changes on a daily basis. In many cases, some people don't want to know all the details, and if he sounds fine, they don't have to deal with it.

"Nobody wants to believe it. We can all be on our best behavior for the moment, though not for long," she explains. It's similar to anyone "holding it all together" during challenging times.

Alisha and Bonnie offer the following nuggets of insight:

▶ *If someone is stressed or ill, they may respond better to non-verbal communication. Sudden noises also throw them off or put them in a hyper-vigilant mode.*

▶ *They may have difficulty hearing every word if their minds easily drift. Sometimes people can shut out or pretend not to hear something because they didn't want to hear it.*

▶ *Body level is another important consideration. Most people, especially those with dementia or memory loss, are uncomfortable if someone is standing above them.*

▶ *Be as specific as possible and avoid pronouns. Leave out unnecessary details and words.*

▶ *Eliminate distractions by involving them in smaller groups.*

▶ *Avoid clichés like "hop in the shower," that they may have trouble understanding.*

▶ *Determine the best time of day for your loved one to talk, do things or go places.*

This theme of communication continues as the caregivers meet with Bonnie who notes that when the clients are together by themselves with the other facilitator, they don't have to work as hard or "be on display." Too many noises and voices in a big group tend to distract individuals with dementia or memory loss. Keep that in mind during the holidays.

One woman says they had a smaller family gathering recently, and her husband said it was much nicer so he could focus better on fewer members.

The new reality for many families coping with Alzheimer's or memory loss is that big family events and certain traditions may become things of the past. It's better for the client and the immediate caregiver to spread the holidays out over a longer period with smaller groups. It takes a lot of energy to participate in a crowd.

"The world will not end if you don't make everybody's favorite cookie. There's always the bakery. It's easier to smile than wear yourself out. It's not worth getting upset more than necessary. Spread out the responsibilities."

The motto, "we've always done it this way" is not permanent anymore, she explains.

One caregiver has created a journal to "dump on the kids" and "bless them with his bad times." However, it's important to balance bad news with good news.

Many families have discovered that sending weekly or monthly updates is good enough to keep everyone informed and make it a reality. No one should later claim that they didn't know or understand. Bonnie suggests that before the holidays, tell everybody what to expect and how changes are necessary. Out-of-towners may have to stay at a hotel this time.

"Some relatives will just not pay attention, but they need to be warned that it won't be the same old thing. Warn them that they may need to prepare for hard decisions." This is just another way to bring reality to those who are still in denial.

At the same time, Bonnie stresses, you don't want the caregiver, often the other parent, to feel embarrassed by the illness. It's nothing they did or can control.

A brother berated the mom for the dad's disease but later apologized.

Bonnie suggests the easiest way to change denial is let the nay-sayer be responsible for the loved one's care for a couple of hours.

"That'll clear it up pretty fast." She smiles.

One mother had her son take his dad out golfing one day. The son quickly discovered what was going on.

"I need to work on my embarrassment. I want to crawl under a rock when Mom yells in the restaurant."

One is angered by relatives who claim to know everything. "You don't know! You aren't here!"

"There is no fixing it. It's a hard realization."

"If only we could be as happy as they are."

Bonnie acknowledges that few disorders and diseases are as hard physically and emotionally on families as Alzheimer's and related conditions. The relationship with this person loses its focus with loss after loss, igniting a grief that may be difficult to identify. It can also create anger at everybody and everything, an urgent feeling that "we have to do something!"

The caregivers notice someone missing this week and wonder if everything is all right. Bonnie reassures the group that she'll call this individual, but uses this opportunity to remind everybody that people need control in their lives to make choices. Some feel bombarded at this stage. Some people feel worse hearing other experiences. "It's sometimes overwhelming."

At her husband's recent birthday party, the wife reports that 90 percent of those in attendance probably think she's got the problem, not him, because he did so well.

One client is having more trouble answering the telephone.

Bonnie suggests getting caller ID and turning off the ringer so that it goes directly to the answering machine. One less stress.

She reminds them that those individuals who didn't routinely ask for assistance before dementia are unlikely to ask for help now.

One says her husband had turned off the water heater pilot light instead of the water when they left for a few days.

"We get frustrated, but it's the disease," Bonnie says. "How do we cope emotionally? We're told to have hope, patience and a sense of humor, but you can't survive if you don't find your own coping methods."

A caregiver told of how she'd left for a few hours, and her loved one was depressed and scared when she returned. The next day, the loved one looked for her frequently for reassurance that she hadn't left again.

"You're the center of her world. Like a young child, what she can't see doesn't exist. It's the same thing with dementia. They know it but forget it."

Another reports it took nearly four hours to get her husband ready to go out. He has several pairs of identical dark sweatpants and white shirts but wanted a certain one and wasn't satisfied until he got it.

One says that their son watched his father search everywhere in the kitchen for the dishwasher. Finally, the son pointed it out. It was a hard fact of life that his father has Alzheimer's.

A spouse had a scary moment when a friend dropped her husband off at the wrong restaurant. Luckily someone there knew him and helped.

Another laments, "I forget that he can't remember."

Bonnie explains that relationships, that once were automatic, aren't anymore. You can't tell them to do something else while they're doing another thing. They often can't handle more than one instruction at a time.

"You get to be human and complain and be afraid. They'll often just sit there and become what we view as apathetic. Are they content to do nothing? They are more than we realize."

If the family is considering adult day care, ask the staff to work with them to create jobs for the individual with dementia or memory loss. Bonnie says the local center is good at finding jobs that give them a sense of purpose and something to do.

"You have to know the person to know if they'll be sociable. And some people are simply non-people persons." However, she cautions that if the family waits too long to get them to interact in an adult day care setting, it may not work at all.

A caregiver says her daughter told her she didn't want the mother "hating" the father because she had assumed sole responsibility for his care and not asked for any help.

"You have to set the stage for communication," Bonnie explains. "You don't want your kids mad at both of you for not getting help. You're making decisions for your daughter because you think she's too busy."

Nods of recognition sweep the room.

Caregivers must pay close attention to their own needs

After listening to and assisting hundreds of families in the last decade at the Alzheimer's Association, education specialist Bonnie says she's heard many clients express concern that their caregivers will endanger their own health when the responsibility becomes too much to handle.

"They were afraid the caregiver would try to keep them at home for longer than they should or are able, to the point where it impacts *their* health."

A lot of caregivers are in their 80s, and excessive stress and physical demands can put their health in jeopardy. Many caregivers would never admit that, or they'll promise that they'll never put them in a nursing home.

"No, *never, never* promise anyone that," she stresses. The focus has to be on everyone's safety, and a worn-out caregiver can't adequately protect someone who is wholly dependent on them.

Caregivers need to look at their own needs from Day 1 as it's a balance between quality of life and safety for both. For some caregivers, they may be able to go the duration.

"What's the caregiver's health situation? It really is a personal thing. Different people can do it so much longer than others. It's based on personal things, physical and emotional strength, patience, and the pre-existing relationship. We're assuming that all those couples married for 60 years were happy. Wrong!"

She smiles.

"I don't think there's anything that it's not okay to ask for help. I tell caregivers that they may need financial, legal or physical help, or they may need spiritual help to reach out if that's always been a part of their life, or in a crisis." Some people question their faith when they're in situations like this. "The spiritual piece is huge in the grief process."

Many lament that it's just not fair, though Bonnie has learned much from the caregiver who simply acknowledges that it's part of life. You don't have to like it, but it just happens.

Caregivers need someone who will listen, listen, listen, she says, and not necessarily try to "fix it" unless the caregiver asks for that advice. That's why some caregivers hesitate talking to family or friends because they know they'll be "told" what to do, i.e., put them in a nursing home. But many will say, "I'll know when I want to do that. I just want them to listen. I just want to be heard."

She learns something new from every family.

"Just seeing how incredibly flexible and patient they can be with their person … How they see it as a challenge, not a burden, even an honor almost. I've come across caregivers like that."

She's found that the more educational programs the Alzheimer's Association offers, the fewer crisis calls they get because many families have their "tools." They pull together and find ways to make positive choices.

The story of a caregiver who didn't run and hide when her husband began singing in the grocery store inspires her.

"She chose to celebrate the sparkle of the man she loves and not be embarrassed. It's the perfect example of how you have a choice. It's not always easy, but how you cope is a choice."

One of her favorite phone calls was from a woman who described how her husband used to work third shift and slept during the daytime, and he kept up that sleeping habit. Bonnie asked if she had contacted the doctor to see if he needed a sleeping aid. But the woman replied that now they both sleep during the day and stay up all night.

Does it surprise caregivers when they find they can cope?

"I don't think they even think about it. They do what they need to do. In retrospective, they say, 'How did I get through all that?' Because you didn't have a choice. Not doing it didn't seem like an option."

How have I been affected?

_____

_____

_____

_____

Caregivers say...

The theory that "if you don't take care of yourself, you can't take care of someone else," has been put to the test again and again for caregivers of dementia and memory loss individuals. The results are usually the same: caregivers *have* to put their own needs first more often if they want to be effective, stay healthy and continuing being their loved one's advocate.

184

How did or do you take care of your own needs?

- Only took care of the basics
- With sitters
- Went to Alzheimer's Association meetings
- Made time for R&R
- Ate well
- Exercised
- Take one day at a time
- Awareness from previous training
- Counseling and medication
- Maintained a balanced life
- Did the necessary things and let the rest go
- By remaining in my own home
- By selling a big house and moving into a condo
- Driving
- Mow my yard
- Gardening
- Reading and writing
- Talk openly with friends and family about my feelings and needs
- Hired part-time housekeeper and caregiver
- Supportive spouse who helped with meals, etc.
- Take him to daughter's house one day a week
- Take him to weekly respite program
- With difficulty and practice
- Volunteered in community
- In-between his needs
- Allowed myself to rest
- I didn't
- Tried to live my life fully
- Pace the workload
- My life revolved around my mom in the nursing home and if they needed to get ahold of me. *Jolene, 66, mother, dementia, died 5 years after diagnosed*

▸ Exercise. I tried to keep up regular activities. I'd bike out to where he lived. I became a workaholic since my work involves developing community service for Alzheimer's. *Ann, 49, mother, vascular dementia, died; father, Alzheimer's, died*

▸ I try to get away for a few hours. I almost always take Mom everywhere I go. When I don't, I feel sad and guilty. *Jenny, 56, mother, Alzheimer's*

▸ I don't always. Sometimes take time for myself, spend time with family and friends. *Mary Ann, 62, father, Alzheimer's*

▸ I can't. I have no income or insurance. *Nettie, 51, father, Alzheimer's*

▸ I'm learning to rest when he naps instead of always trying to get chores done. *Helen, 72, husband, Alzheimer's*

▸ My sisters usually took her on weekends, usually willingly. *Darlene, 58, mother, Alzheimer's*

▸ I don't think you really do, but I took time weekly for myself. *Gayle, 59, mother, Alzheimer's, died 5 years after diagnosed*

▸ My mom doesn't get out enough. I try to stop by most mornings for coffee after my child's at school, just so she has another adult to talk to. *Mary, 38, father, Alzheimer's*

▸ I cry and then go on. *Chris, 51, mother, Alzheimer's*

▸ I make sure I use makeup and do my hair and dress each morning so I will be ready for any emergency. I take my medication and eat well. *Norma, 81, husband, Alzheimer's*

How can I take care of me?

Professionals say...

Healthcare professionals are people, too.

How are you affected by your work emotionally and physically? How do you cope with that?

▶ I become emotionally involved because you care for these clients at least five days a week. *Latoya, 27, CNA, 2 years*

▶ I love my work, my residents. I care for them so much. I am tired at the end of the day but am happy with what I do. *Kalah, 48, social service assistant, four months*

▶ I have developed coping mechanisms. *Dave, 40, executive director, 2 years*

▶ Yes, you become attached, but I try to remember I made a difference in that person's end-of-life years. *Cindy, 53, nurse, 34 years*

▶ I have a best friend who is my support! *Marge, 50, nursing home administrator, 24 years*

▶ Emotional attachment, the patient dying. Physical abuse to staff that comes with Alzheimer's. Physical, realizing patient is not his/herself. *Sherry, 27, trainer, 2 years*

▶ Sometimes drained from both staff and participant issues. I use a peer or supervisor for sounding block. *Ronni, R.N, 49, 28 years*

▶ I get very attached and when I lose a patient, it hurts. I give hugs to others. *Sharon, 55, nurse aide/driver, 15 years*

▶ I try not to absorb the emotions. Sitting too long hurts my body. I lift weights, go horseback riding, have great friends. *Connie, 57, psychotherapist*

▶ The most difficult part is lack of interest in family members. I cope by trying to be there more for the patient. *Michelle, 48, CNA, 30 years*

▶ Tired, happy. Hobbies help. *Trudy, 57, director of nursing, 30 years*

▶ I have to take time off work to take my husband to doctors appointments. I cannot stay to get my work done, because I have to pick him up at a set time. I'm having to work at home just to get the bills paid. *Gloria, 54, CNA, 18 years*

▶ I am bothered when families are not happy. I try to go above and beyond to meet their needs. *Susan, 38, R.N., 12 years*

▶ It's not about me. I don't know if I cope well or not. *Karen, 46, developmental technician, 20 years*

▶ Seeing someone decline, it's not easy, but I don't show the concern in my face, so they do not get upset. *Debi, 48, trainer, 6 years*

▶ We laugh at work. Good relationship with my co-workers. *Mary, 37, hospital social worker, 11 years*

▶ I enjoy my work but do feel physically and emotionally drained due to a hyperactive physical resident. *Susan, 58, LPN*

What can I learn from others?

Caregivers say...

Every caregiver should have reservoirs of emotional or physical outlets to get through the tough times.

188 What was the most useful thing that has helped you maintain your strength during caregiving?

- Help from others
- Knowledge
- Family support
- Prayer and faith
- Church
- Love
- Laughter
- Alzheimer's Association
- Respite care
- Knowing I could get away for a few hours
- Patience with myself
- Knowing "this too shall pass"
- Adult day care center
- Psychiatrist
- Therapist
- Online support group
- Clinical mindset
- Support group meetings
- His nap in the afternoon
- Outside activities
- Doctors
- Friends
- Advice of other caregivers
- Spirituality
- Grieving as needed
- Love and care at nursing home
- Love and respect for my husband
- Loving memories of Mom

- Thankful for the opportunity to spend time before the end came. *Sylvia, 58, mother, Alzheimer's, died 17 years after diagnosed*

- Making sure we had our away time. Taking care of yourself is a must. *John, 67, mother-in-law, Alzheimer's*

- Giving Mom a few good years of enjoyment. *Jenny, 56, mother, Alzheimer's*

" My husband's support and humor." Ellen, 69, mother

▶ Getting relief from adult day care and then having a live-in caregiver so my mom could live in her own home. *Jolene, 66, mother, dementia, died 5 years after diagnosed*

▶ Knowledgeable friends and caregivers, understanding boss and family. *Ann, 49, mother, vascular dementia, died; father, Alzheimer's, died*

▶ Talking to other co-workers/friends who are experiencing the same thing. *Cathi, 58, mother, dementia*

▶ Knowing that I could give back to Dad the love and support he gave me. *Mary Ann, 62, father, Alzheimer's*

▶ Prayer, sense of humor, not thinking of me. If you think of yourself, you had better quit. *Robert, 79, wife, Alzheimer's, died 6 years after diagnosed*

▶ Visiting frequently, giving her little gifts. *Ann, 63, aunt, Alzheimer's, died 6 years after diagnosed*

> "The nursing home staff, friends and the ability to separate myself from it."
> Nancy, 65, mother, Alzheimer's

▶ Praying to God for strength and believing in myself to do the job. *Shirley, 72, husband, dementia*

▶ Support of my husband and two sisters. If they lived close by, we could have shared Mom's care and perhaps she could have lived with one of us. That was not possible in our current situation. *Judith, 61, mother, Alzheimer's*

▶ Love of friends and family expressed in caring and thoughtful actions. *Anne, 67, mother, dementia, died 4 years after diagnosed*

▶ My children and recognizing that I may need them to care for me some day. *Elizabeth, 47, mother, Alzheimer's*

▶ I know that my mom joined a support group of women in similar situations, which was extremely helpful for her. *Andrew, 25, father, frontal lobe dementia, diagnosed at age 51*

▶ Grace of God. We can't do this without help. *Mary, 38, father, Alzheimer's*

There are no stereotypes

Greg is that stereotypical perfect picture of health and vitality. He exercises regularly, eats properly, is hard-working, intelligent, generous, a dad, brother to six siblings, in his early 50s and savoring life with great enthusiasm every day.

He has everything he wants and something he doesn't want … early-onset Alzheimer's.

Attired in running shorts and shoes, Greg prepares to lead the crowd at the annual fall Alzheimer's Association Memory Walk. The gorgeous sky and hot sun make it more like summer than autumn, and that brings out hundreds of supporters who vow to walk for those who can't and those who are here in spirit only. They all have a common goal: *end Alzheimer's disease.*

You'd never imagine that behind the stylish eyeglass frames and beneath the closely trimmed haircut is a man who's battling early-onset Alzheimer's with every source of energy he's got. He had a good life working in Chicago as an accountant, never missing a day of work. Then he noticed some memory problems that were beginning to affect his work.

His doctor referred him for an MRI, where the technician told him, "Take it one day at a time." He laughs at that memory before his world flipped upside down with the diagnosis.

"One day at a time … That's all I do. What I have stinks, but that's what I have to deal with. I'm reconciled with it. This is my plight. This is what I have to do. I still get up every morning, still work and drive. That may be a problem at one point. I'm sure it will be. Other than that, I'm doing good, I'm in great shape, I've got a great family. When the news came down, they were all around me. No ifs, ands or buts. They got me down here."

That support system includes four sisters and two brothers, who grew up in a tiny house where the girls shared one bedroom and the boys the attic. After the memory symptoms snowballed, he admits he couldn't deal with it and moved back home to be close to family.

His siblings offer substantial emotional, physical and financial support as he copes with unexpected life changes, having to find work that didn't tax his memory skills too much. It's not the most exciting job in the world, but "I'm doing something."

Despite everything, he says, "I couldn't be in a better situation."

Is it hard for him to ask for help?

"I haven't got to that point yet, but I probably will sometime. Nobody knows. It's just the circle of life. It's a tough thing not knowing what's going to happen or how fast it's going to go."

A few months earlier, he traveled to Washington, D.C., to offer testimony on the need for additional funding and to show the world that Alzheimer's does not claim only the elderly.

"Just get some money. That's what we need. I feel like I'm contributing something. I feel like I'm helping some people ..."

Greg is certainly not the voice or face one would expect to help kick-off the annual walk as the growing crowd listens ...

"My name is Greg, and I was diagnosed a year and a half ago." He pauses. "Hold on. I'm having a Greg moment here and need to stop for a moment."

"It's okay," a female voice calls out. He smiles.

"I have to deal with this every day of my life. It's tough, but I don't dwell on it. I'm doing the best I can, and I've got a great family. They're helping me tremendously, and I can't thank them enough. I'm doing all right now, but I don't know what the future holds ..."

Three of Greg's sisters cheer him on from the crowd, so proud of their brother who has refused to hide from the world and who has vowed to make a difference any way he can.

What changes did they witness in him over time?

His temperament changed ... he wasn't as social as he used to be ... he'd leave without warning at family gatherings ... he couldn't understand games he had played all his life.

No wonder they wondered what was happening. Speculation on the cause ranged from a stroke to depression to adult ADD, for which he was prescribed medication.

He lived with one sister who observed that it took him hours to read the newspaper. He needed a job, but he couldn't comprehend the application process. The family pushed and encouraged him, and he kept saying, "I'm not stupid."

As the family gathered to absorb the news of the diagnosis, they remembered how Greg at first thought it was a death sentence. He started talking about where he wanted to be buried. He was concerned about his two adult children.

He wants to be at his daughter's wedding, and his family has vowed, "He will."

191

Caregivers say...

Many caregivers are blessed to have supportive family members and friends, while others wonder if anyone is listening to them ... or even cares.

192

How did friends and other family members respond to changes required to care for this person?

▸ They don't care

▸ They hardly come around

▸ Responsibilities fell to me

▸ Very helpful and patient

▸ There's no other family

▸ Took them years to accept the situation

▸ Mostly understanding

▸ One child is greatest help

▸ Friends became distant

▸ They didn't understand

▸ Offered support

▸ Kept up communication

▸ Friends more supportive than family

▸ Not much of a change ... so far

▸ They weren't very understanding in some cases. Others are now beginning to understand how demanding and difficult it is. *Christl, 55, father, stroke and Alzheimer's*

▸ They understood and were very thoughtful, especially when she walked out in the neighborhood wearing only a slip. *Sylvia, 58, mother, Alzheimer's, died 17 years after diagnosed*

▸ Exceptionally well. My (teenagers) helped a lot, were very patient and developed great compassion, patience and respect for elders. *Ann, 49, mother, vascular dementia, died; father, Alzheimer's, died*

▸ I was the sole caregiver. Other residents in the apartment complex helped her find her way to the dining room, etc. *Judith, 61, mother, Alzheimer's*

"Every family member had to become accustomed to her new way of life."
Shallen, 25, grandmother, Alzheimer's

▸ Several friends have stopped doing things with us. We used to golf. Now he and I go on good days. We don't keep score, and he can still hit the ball. *Pat, 66, husband, Alzheimer's*

▸ Everyone has bonded to get through this. We're very fortunate. It doesn't always happen. *Laurie, 47, father, dementia*

▸ Saying a nursing home is better. They do not feel that way now. *John, 67, mother-in-law, Alzheimer's*

▸ Three adult children share responsibility. Half of adult grandchildren tend to be in denial. *Cathi, 58, mother, dementia*

▸ Friends, as well as family members, expressed what a burden it was. *Jenny, 56, mother, Alzheimer's*

▸ Friends were good. Brothers resisted, ignored, stayed away, avoided, denied. *Chris, 51, mother, Alzheimer's*

▸ Adjusted accordingly. My brother and sister-in-law share equally in the responsibilities. *Mary Ann, 62, father, Alzheimer's*

▸ My family all had their own affairs to care for. They were there if I needed them. A couple of friends stayed close. *Robert, 79, wife, Alzheimer's, died 6 years after diagnosed*

▸ Fantastically! My children and adult grandchildren were totally supportive and helpful. *Anne, 67, mother, dementia, died 4 years after diagnosed*

▸ They did nothing. I could talk or vent to them, but that was all. *Elaine, 54, mother, Alzheimer's*

▸ Some urged me to bring her to my house. I could not do that. My marriage came first! *Nancy, 65, mother, Alzheimer's*

▸ Our son and one daughter became very emotionally available. Both have stayed with Dad so I could get out alone. *Marlene, 68, husband, dementia/Alzheimer's*

▸ My brother has been fantastic. We have gotten super close. *Kevin, 45, mother, Alzheimer's*

"A neighbor quit speaking to me, thinking I should have not put him in the nursing home." *Edna, 83, husband, Alzheimer's, died 7 years after diagnosed*

▸ I wasn't able to do a lot with my friends or family, especially the last year and a half. I stayed home, and Mom took top priority. My husband was very supportive. I think it was hardest on my son. Grandma was mean to him, and it was hard for him to understand. One of Mom's friends wouldn't call her on the phone anymore but would call me. It was because Mom repeated herself a lot. *MM, 46, mother, Alzheimer's, died 5 years after diagnosed*

▸ With sympathy. Friends wouldn't visit him when he was living alone. He had to go bowling or to church, etc., to see them. *Marcy, 76, father, Alzheimer's, died 5 years after diagnosed*

▸ It is hard on my husband and children since they've had to change their lifestyle and give their time. My siblings act as if she is already dead. *Elizabeth, 47, mother, Alzheimer's*

▸ There was some anger, the thought that she was beyond caring or knowing, so "why bother?" *Kim, 34, grandmother, died 5 years after diagnosed*

▸ I am blessed. While in our home, it was a little tense, but I was free to do whatever, and my spouse kept the home life going. *Gayle, 59, mother, Alzheimer's, died 5 years after diagnosed*

▸ Some stopped coming because of his actions and not being able to converse. *Catherine, 85, husband, Alzheimer's and Lewy Body*

▸ Most didn't know what to do or what to say. It is hard to understand how someone my dad's age could come down with something so unlikely. *Andrew, 25, father, frontal lobe dementia, diagnosed at age 51*

▸ One brother pulled away completely. Most friends pulled away. One brother lived in another state but called regularly, and one brother relieved me one week. *Sally, 57, mother, Alzheimer's, died 3 years after diagnosed*

▸ Mostly family pulled together to get things done. I have been disappointed by my parents' church friends who said they'd help, but it never happened. *Mary, 38, father, Alzheimer's*

▸ All offered to help. He refuses anyone coming into our home but does go to our daughters' homes one day a week. *Sandy, 61, husband, Alzheimer's and vascular dementia*

Caregivers say...

It's not easy to ask for help, and sometimes it's not easy to offer help. However, while most caregivers are reluctant to ask for help, they will most often accept specific gestures of assistance.

Did they offer assistance without being asked or only upon request?

▶ They generally ask

▶ Yes

▶ No

▶ On request

▶ Without being asked

▶ They made suggestions

▶ A little of both

▶ They just don't understand

▶ Some did, some didn't

▶ Offered but didn't help

▶ Without being asked; they also offered money and time to give me a break. *Sylvia, 58, mother, Alzheimer's, died 17 years after diagnosed*

▶ Everybody helps when possible. *Cathi, 58, mother, dementia*

▶ One sister-in-law was so good to go along, but another refused to go. *Norma, 81, mother, Alzheimer's, died 11 years after diagnosed; sister, Alzheimer's, died 6 years after diagnosed*

▶ I've had no problems. *Maxine, 77, husband, Alzheimer's*

▶ Our daughter did help when asked. *Robert, 79, wife, Alzheimer's, died 6 years after diagnosed*

▶ There were no other family members here to help. One sister took Mom to her home for a week a couple of times a year until it became too hard on Mom. *Judith, 61, mother, Alzheimer's*

▶ Just advice, not all good. *Nancy, 65, mother, Alzheimer's*

"Family offered. Friends were uncomfortable. Golf buddies vanished." *Marcy, 76, husband, memory loss due to massive stroke*

▶ Upon request. My kids are all supportive, though I think the one most like him was in denial for a long time. I didn't let them know how bad things were for a long time. I was trying to spare them and protect their dad's dignity. I did that a lot. *Marlene, 68, husband, dementia/ Alzheimer's*

▶ It depends on their personality. One sibling sees need and fills it. Other two want to help but need direction. *Mary, 38, father, Alzheimer's*

Did you feel comfortable asking for help? Why?

▶ From doctors and staff

▶ Typically for my mom

▶ Sometimes

▶ Sometimes it was awkward

▶ No, it was my place to take care of him

▶ Yes, because Dad's well-being was my top concern

▶ Not especially because I was used to doing things for myself

▶ Yes, because I knew I couldn't do it alone

▶ Asked for help and got it as needed

▶ Only when it became necessary

▶ I didn't want to inconvenience anyone

▶ I didn't at first but realized my friends wanted to help

▶ No, because I didn't want to hear lame excuses why they could not help

▶ No, because of resistance though it got better

▶ Sometimes now. I feel like I'm supposed to cope on my own and that I am a failure if I ask for help. *Christl, 55, father, stroke and Alzheimer's*

▶ Yes, because it's very stressful, and no, because that's my grandma. *Shallen, 25, grandmother, Alzheimer's*

▶ Yes. It's important not to do everything alone. *John, 67, mother-in-law, Alzheimer's*

▶ I never asked for help. They weren't able to do anything. *Jolene, 66, mother, dementia, died 5 years after diagnosed*

▶ Yes. Caring for two parents, two kids and husband is a huge responsibility, and there was no one else. *Ann, 49, mother, vascular dementia, died; father, Alzheimer's, died*

▸ We are a family and that is what family does for each other. *Cathi, 58, mother, dementia, diagnosed*

▸ No, because none of them wanted the responsibility of caring for her. It would have made little difference to them if she was in a nursing home. *Jenny, 56, mother, Alzheimer's*

▸ No, I felt he needed me close especially toward the end. *Roseann, 72, husband, dementia, died 10 years after diagnosed*

▸ Yard now done by neighbors. Handy man needs income. Family is great and expects to be asked. *Maxine, 77, husband, Alzheimer's*

▸ People would rather not be bothered, it seems. *David, 69, wife, Alzheimer's*

▸ I didn't have to ask my sister. We planned together, dismantled Dad's house and furnishings, sold the house. But I was the "on-site" person. *Marcy, 76, father, Alzheimer's, died 5 years after diagnosed*

▸ I lived five miles from Mom, worked part-time in the town she lived in, and my husband was a tremendous help. I didn't need to ask for help. *Judith, 61, mother, Alzheimer's*

▸ Yes, we have mutual respect for each other's needs. *Anne, 67, mother, dementia, died 4 years after diagnosed*

▸ Sometimes. I try not to overburden my husband and children since they already give a lot. *Elizabeth, 47, mother, Alzheimer's*

▸ No, but that is a life-long affliction of mine. *Kim, 34, grandmother, died 5 years after diagnosed*

▸ Yes and no. I'm a control freak. I knew it would be done right if I was doing it. *Gayle, 59, mother, Alzheimer's, diagnosed 1997, died 2002*

▸ My husband was not allowed to come home until help was arranged. Visiting nurse kept track of his needs monthly. *Marcy, 76, husband, memory loss due to massive stroke*

▸ No, it was hard for my brother to take time off work. He didn't deal with it easily. *Jody, 47, mother, early onset Alzheimer's*

▸ No, I enjoy doing things myself. I never know how my husband will react to people who come by. *Catherine, 85, husband, Alzheimer's and Lewy Body*

▸ She refused help other than from me. *Bill, 78, wife, Alzheimer's, died 4 years after diagnosed*

▸ They needed to understand how much work it is and how bad she is deteriorating. *Brian, 47, mother, Alzheimer's*

▸ Yes, it is a team effort. You must do it together, or the one doing it will drop of exhaustion. Maybe it's easier for me to ask for help for my caregiver mother than if I were the caregiver. *Mary, 38, father, Alzheimer's*

▸ No, I was afraid to interrupt others' lives. I would also be hurt if they refused. I had family members who helped for a while but complained the whole time. Other members I didn't want to help, because it was not in my mom's best interests. Also my mom would have been embarrassed for people to see her like she was. *MM, 46, mother, Alzheimer's, died 5 years after diagnosed*

What's easiest to ask for?

_____
_____
_____

What am I afraid to ask?

_____
_____
_____

Dealing with those relatives who aren't involved or who just don't "get it"

How should families get past anger and resentment toward members' inability or unwillingness to be involved?

"Every family deals with it in a different way," says Bonnie, an Alzheimer's Association education specialist. The family must look realistically at what needs to be done, at what people are able to do and what skills they possess.

There are some people who just can't help with personal care, but they could mow the lawn. Maybe it's filling in during a primary caregiver's vacation. Maybe it's running errands.

Be upfront when talking about the needs and challenges facing the family. Sometimes it's just being the sounding board. Some family members have helped out more than they ever expected because of their location. She hears more frustration from families where everybody lives in town but who don't or won't help.

"My advice to them is stop wasting *your* energy on a lost cause. They're the ones, who aren't involved, who I really believe will be sorry down the road for not being around while they could still create connections and help."

She tells primary caregivers, so they can't be accused later of not informing everybody, to use e-mail to tell what's going on this week or this month or here's what the doctor said.

"If they answer or ask anything, that's great. If not, they're not going to later say, 'Why didn't you tell me …' If they're not willing to help, they don't get to vote, or maybe not that harshly, but pretty much. My new rule is that is what caller ID is for. If you're not in the mood to deal with them, then don't answer the phone."

One caregiver encountered constant frustration in communicating with her sister who lived out of town. The sister was in denial about any problem with their mother, who had been diagnosed with Alzheimer's. The mother was "just fine" when the sister talked to her, so she asked, "what is the big deal?"

Another caregiver explains that "some people think writing a check will take care of everything. It doesn't solve all the problems."

How you can build your team without screaming

You're frustrated, exhausted, short-tempered, ignored and a multitude of other aggravating verbs.

And let's throw in a few other descriptive terms ... resentful, impatient, forgotten, empty ... alone.

Okay, now that you've acknowledged all that, breathe.

It's time to create *your* caregiving team, the team that's going to support *you* during the time you're devoted to caring for your loved one with dementia or memory loss.

Yes, it may seem easier to ask for assistance from relatives who live nearby or within a couple hundred miles. However, the ones right down the street may be the least interested or involved. The ones who live thousands of miles away may be quite eager to help, though the distance makes it difficult.

It's time to explore the questions you need to ask yourself about the involvement of other family members or friends.

The best and most objective approach may be the creation of a list of talents and hobbies. When you call upon someone for assistance, think first of their availability, skills and things they like to do. Use this as an opportunity to encourage them to put their knowledge to use in a new and positive way.

Don't call it a chore. Don't call it work. Don't call it a responsibility. Foremost, don't call it an obligation or say "You owe me."

Many people consider a gift as something material, something they can hold in their hands and unwrap. Learn how to redefine the word "gift" as something given from the hearts, hands and minds of family or friends, without any damage to their wallets.

However, we all know individuals who only know how to write checks. They may feel uncomfortable showing emotion or being around someone with dementia or memory loss who may no longer remember them. They honestly do not know what to say or do, and nothing you say or do will change their insecurities and fears. Do not subject yourself to the aggravation of repeatedly asking for anything else beyond financial assistance.

It takes tremendous courage to ask for help. The fear of rejection is enormous, intense and even paralyzing at times. Some people are so stubborn that they'd rather die first than ask for assistance.

Unfortunately, there are caregivers who have died first after working themselves into an exhausted state or not taken care of their own physical, emotional and medical needs and refused help.

And where does that leave your loved one?

Put your team together *today*.

Questions to ask yourself   201

If and when you need to involve more family members in the caregiving of a loved one with dementia or memory loss, exam all the possible opportunities. Consider using these questions to build upon while creating your own list and where local and out-of-town relatives and friends may be able to assist. Think of the everyday responsibilities you have in caregiving and add those.

▸ *Who has time to help me?*

▸ *Who has any Sunday morning, noon or night of the month free?*

▸ *Who has any Monday morning, noon or night of the month free?*

▸ *Who has any Tuesday morning, noon or night of the month free?*

▸ *Who has any Wednesday morning, noon or night of the month free?*

▸ *Who has any Thursday morning, noon or night of the month free?*

▸ *Who has any Friday morning, noon or night of the month free?*

▸ *Who has any Saturday morning, noon or night of the month free?*

▸ *Who has the financial resources to help me?*

▸ *Who could help pay for in-home care to give me a break day or night?*

▸ *Who could spend a week or weekend with my loved one so I could take a vacation?*

▸ *Who has the physical strength to help me?*

▸ *Who could I ask to help move some furniture around to make every-thing more convenient for me and/or my loved one?*

▸ *Who could take my loved one for a walk?*

▸ *Who could take my loved one out for coffee?*

▸ *Who could take my loved one for a drive?*

▸ *Who could stay with my loved one for a short time while I run errands?*

▶ Who loves to clean?

▶ Who is the expert organizer of paperwork?

▶ Who is the expert organizer of clothing and personal items?

▶ Who could sort through items like books or magazines to give to a charitable garage sale?

▶ Who could clean and organize kitchen cabinets and pantries?

▶ Who loves to bake sweets?

▶ Who loves to prepare meals?

▶ Who makes my favorite soup?

▶ Who could go grocery shopping for me?

▶ Who could pick up fresh fruits and vegetables at the farmers' market?

▶ Who could pick up my favorite restaurant meal?

▶ Who could pick up DVDs at the video store?

▶ Who could pick up some books or magazines at the book store?

▶ Who is the expert handyperson for the inside house maintenance?

▶ Who is the expert handyperson for the outside house maintenance?

▶ Who could pick up salt for the water softener and pour it in?

▶ Who could contact professionals for more complex maintenance and repair needs?

▶ Who loves to garden?

▶ Who could plant some flowers around the yard?

▶ Who could make a small window box of flowers for my loved one to see, touch and smell?

▶ Who could mow the yard?

▶ Who could pull weeds and clear away other landscape waste?

▶ Who could make sure outdoor plants are watered regularly?

▶ Who could clean out the garage?

▶ Who could organize tools or other items that are in disarray?

▶ Who has a friendly pet to bring by to entertain?

▶ Who has younger children who could practice their reading skills by reading to your loved one?

▸ Who has younger children who could engage your loved one in activities like coloring, playing dominos, etc.?

▸ Who tells funny stories?

▸ Who is a great listener?

▸ Who will give me time to vent?

▸ Who will give me time to cry?

▸ Who will give me a hug?

▸ Who will tell me they love me?

My who's who list

Caregivers say...

At one time or another, we're not sure what to say or do when someone we know is going through a difficult situation. Sometimes they need some suggestions to do or say "the right thing."

Sometimes people don't know what to say or do. What did others say or do to help you during your process of caregiving that was helpful?

- Shared personal experiences
- Encouraged to attend support group
- "It will get better"
- Friend sent encouraging e-mails daily
- Friends visited occasionally
- Friends took us out to eat
- Asked how they could help
- Church friends gave comfort

- Nothing
- Concerned
- Supportive
- Friends inquired frequently how I was doing
- Most praised us for what we were doing
- Not much was said
- "You're a good daughter"
- "Can I help?"
- "Call anytime you need us"

- Just acknowledging how difficult and draining that it can be and that I'm not alone in the world doing this. *Christl, 55, father, stroke and Alzheimer's*

- Be honest. Say what's on your mind. Let it out so it doesn't build up and you explode. *Laurie, 47, father, dementia*

- "I don't know how you do it" or "She's lucky to have you guys," but not much help. *John, 67, mother-in-law, Alzheimer's*

- My husband was wonderful and helped all the time. He was very close to my mother. *Jolene, 66, mother, dementia, died 5 years after diagnosed*

- Send cards and letters to my mother. *Phil, 69, mother, dementia*

"Listen to me." Ellen, 69, mother

▸ It reminded me of things I knew as a nurse, but forgot as a caregiver, like introducing myself to my dad after he got to the point he forgot. *Ann, 49, mother, vascular dementia, died; father, Alzheimer's, died*

▸ He has been good at covering up his condition, so I've been told, "He seems good, seems to be okay." Only those who know the disease know what I'm talking about. *Pat, 66, husband, Alzheimer's*

▸ Occasionally my brother needs a reminder. We channel requests through his wife who gets it done! Her grandmother had Alzheimer's. *Cathi, 58, mother, dementia*

▸ My husband has been my only source of comfort. You are right. People don't know what to say or do. *Jenny, 56, mother, Alzheimer's*

▸ The pastor visited Mother, and if I was there when he came, he put me at ease as to how things were. The house was such a mess, and I could do nothing about it. *Norma, 81, mother, Alzheimer's, died 11 years after diagnosed; sister, Alzheimer's, died 6 years after diagnosed*

▸ People don't know, so they would look at me and talk and ignore him. I didn't like that. *Roseann, 72, husband, dementia, died 10 years after diagnosed*

▸ They just tell me it's going to get worse, so take care of myself and call when I need help. *Maxine, 77, husband, Alzheimer's*

▸ I'm not the main caregiver, but physical help is great. I love it when my brother does maintenance we can't handle. Mom always wished some other men would take Dad for walks regularly. It never happened. *Mary, 38, father, Alzheimer's*

▸ Those who came treated her as if she were normal. She would ask them to leave, even family. *Robert, 79, wife, Alzheimer's, died 6 years after diagnosed*

"The most helpful is the head nurse at the Alzheimer's unit since she tells me what to expect next." Elizabeth, 47, mother, Alzheimer's

▸ Help came from support group. Suggestions from their experiences were more beneficial than sympathy. *Marcy, 76, father, Alzheimer's, died 5 years after diagnosed*

▸ They fixed meals and sat with her so I could leave. They offered to do specifics instead of asking what was needed. *Anne, 67, mother, dementia, died 4 years after diagnosed*

▸ Most do not know what to say or do. You are in it alone. *Shirley, 72, husband, dementia*

▸ My close friends often inquired about Mom because their parents are about the same age. *Judith, 61, mother, Alzheimer's*

▸ Some have let me know they are available whenever I need them. Some can't deal with the whole issue. Some have cried with me and laughed with me. Those are the gems. The ones who let you "hurt" in front of them. *Marlene, 68, husband, dementia/Alzheimer's*

▸ Take him some place without my asking. *June, 66, husband, early onset Alzheimer's*

▸ General support, comments from friends, but if you have not lived it, you cannot comprehend it. *Gayle, 59, mother, Alzheimer's, died 5 years after diagnosed*

▸ Towards the end, they would call more often and offer to sit with us. A few would bring meals to me. *Vicky, 54, husband, early onset Alzheimer's, died 5 years after diagnosed*

▸ Often times it was most important or helpful when people told us that they couldn't necessarily understand how to help, but were willing to do anything we asked. *Andrew, 25, father, frontal lobe dementia, diagnosed at age 51*

▸ Mostly by being good listeners. My daughter found a new doctor who has been most helpful. *Martha, 71, husband, cognitive decline*

▸ It was only after she was in a nursing home that I found a weekly support group. *Bill, 78, wife, Alzheimer's, died 4 years after diagnosed*

"Gifts of time or suggestions 'to care for the caregiver' were helpful." *Kim, 34, grandmother, died 5 years after diagnosed*

▶ My nurse friends were very supportive and understanding. Others in the community offer, "I'm so sorry." *Sandy, 61, husband, Alzheimer's and vascular dementia*

▶ "Remember, this isn't your mom. It's the disease." *Jody, 47, mother, early onset Alzheimer's*

▶ They would pray for me. One friend came over with cookies to visit. One brother helped by caring for her one week so I could visit friends in Florida. It was hard to come home! *MM, 46, mother, Alzheimer's, died 5 years after diagnosed*

Who's been helpful so far?

_____

_____

_____

How and why?

_____

_____

_____

_____

Caregivers say...

Human beings aren't perfect. Occasionally and unintentionally, we speak before thinking or offer advice without fully understanding what a caregiver is experiencing. However, some people are simply clueless.

208

Sometimes people say or do things that are hurtful during this time period. What would you advise people NOT to do or say to caregivers?

▸ How your loved one is a burden

▸ How there's no cure

▸ It's not "her" anymore

▸ Imply I should be doing more

▸ Recommend drugs

▸ Don't tell them what to do

▸ Pretend that nothing has changed

▸ "Oh, we all get forgetful"

▸ "I know what it's like"

▸ Forget platitudes

▸ Not following through on offers of assistance

▸ Giving advice when they have no idea what's going on

▸ Don't engage in long conversations the individual can't understand

▸ Don't come late or stay late

▸ Point out "stupid" things he does

▸ Don't offer advice if you've not been through the experience

▸ Don't tell someone that they're wasting their time or life

▸ To insinuate that there is nothing to it, that there is no skill, or that it's not an important job. *Christl, 55, father, stroke and Alzheimer's*

▸ Don't show your frustrations and don't tell the person they are wrong. Just agree with things. *Shallen, 25, grandmother, Alzheimer's*

▸ To say a nursing home is the answer. It is sometimes, but they do need love and hugs. *John, 67, mother-in-law, Alzheimer's*

- Unless they truly understand our situation, they should not say things that make him feel like a dummy. He is not an idiot. *Pat, 66, husband, Alzheimer's*

- Don't pretend that you don't know what is going on. "I can't go in that dirty place. I might throw up." *Norma, 81, mother, Alzheimer's, died 11 years after diagnosed; sister, Alzheimer's, died 6 years after diagnosed*

- I feel like my judgment comes into question with some friends. I have a better understanding of the situation than they do. I live it. *Jenny, 56, mother, Alzheimer's*

- "You mean you don't get paid for this? I couldn't do it." They don't help out but call to tell you what you should do. *Nettie, 51, father, Alzheimer's*

- I didn't pay much attention to them. I guess, consider the source. I guess they're concerned about their problems, not that you're hurting or whatever. Everyone has enough to think of without yours. *Robert, 79, wife, Alzheimer's, died 6 years after diagnosed*

- Focus on supporting their decisions. *Ann, 63, aunt, Alzheimer's, died 6 years after diagnosed*

- I really didn't experience this. I always appreciated people who inquired about Mom. It helps me to talk to others. *Judith, 61, mother, Alzheimer's*

- "You know it is only going to get worse." Caregivers know that. We don't need to be told. *Elaine, 54, mother, Alzheimer's*

- Asking the person to take on more than they can do. *Nancy, 65, mother, Alzheimer's*

- Suggest a nursing home before caregiver is ready. Complaining about how useless their husband is, "he doesn't do anything!" *Marlene, 68, husband, dementia/Alzheimer's*

"Friends of caregivers should keep in touch. A phone call, a visit can mean a lot." Roseann, 72, husband, dementia, died 10 years after diagnosed

▶ No guilt. Let them do what they feel they need to do. *Kim, 34, grandmother, died 5 years after diagnosed*

▶ Do not say, "I understand." They don't! *Vicky, 54, husband, early onset Alzheimer's, died 5 years after diagnosed*

▶ To a certain extent, you don't want to wallow in self-pity and often it isn't helpful to constantly say things like "I don't know how you do it" or "I feel so sorry for you" or "I don't think I could do it." *Andrew, 25, father, frontal lobe dementia, diagnosed at age 51*

▶ Not believing them, blaming the caregiver for the patient's situation. *Brian, 47, mother, Alzheimer's*

▶ People were mostly apathetic rather than hurtful. *Bill, 78, wife, Alzheimer's, died 4 years after diagnosed*

▶ "Why don't you just go, get out!" Well, it's not that simple. *Sandy, 61, husband, Alzheimer's and vascular dementia*

▶ Don't offer to help because the caregiver won't want to bother you. Just show up and allow the caregiver to leave and get away for a while. It's harder to refuse someone when they're already there. *MM, 46, mother, Alzheimer's, died 5 years after diagnosed*

What really hurts me?

_____

_____

_____

_____

_____

_____

Caregivers say...

What do you wish someone would have said or done during this period that was not said or done?

▸ Offer to sit with him so I could get away

▸ Visited more often

▸ Life-long friends should have visited her

▸ "How can I help?"

▸ Offered to take my husband out for coffee or a ride

▸ Just recognize that this is a huge undertaking

▸ Believed me

▸ Taken the time to learn more

▸ "I'll pray for you"

▸ "I'll pick you up"

▸ Thank you for taking on this responsibility, acknowledging how much of your life you give up. *Christl, 55, father, stroke and Alzheimer's*

▸ Be honest! How to cope with anger and different personality (she began cursing), not to agitate her. *Sylvia, 58, mother, Alzheimer's, died 17 years after diagnosed*

▸ We are lucky to be able to say that most things said and done are always positive. *John, 67, mother-in-law, Alzheimer's*

▸ Realize that there is still joy in life when they find things to celebrate, a significant connection or conversation, even if that conversation doesn't always make sense. Don't worry about it. Respond to the feeling of what is said, not the words. *Ann, 49, mother, vascular dementia, died; father, Alzheimer's, died*

▸ Just help out more so I could exercise or get pampered. I have no health insurance now and don't get to go to the doctor. *Nettie, 51, father, Alzheimer's*

"Someone to just give me a long hug." Elaine, 54, mother, Alzheimer's

- One doctor told me "things were not that bad yet." I think doctors could have been more caring. It could have helped me cope and understand the changes. *Pat, 66, husband, Alzheimer's*

- I wish my daughters had said, "I'm sorry Mom that you are slowly losing your mother." *Cathi, 58, mother, dementia*

- I wish my five siblings would be more involved. I used to have things I did, too. *Jenny, 56, mother, Alzheimer's*

- I never thought much about it. The words from family and a couple of friends seemed to help, "I love you." *Robert, 79, wife, Alzheimer's, died 6 years after diagnosed*

- Take her for anything so I could be alone. *David, 69, wife, Alzheimer's*

- No one warned me that I would have to forget rejoining the social world, that caregiving marks you in a way that frightened unaffected people. But saying so would seem unkind. *Marcy, 76, husband, memory loss due to massive stroke*

- I wish my pastor would have overcome his discomfort of ministering to her and would have visited more. He only came twice in two and a half years. *Anne, 67, mother, dementia, died 4 years after diagnosed*

- At first, my brother and sister, who don't live here, did not believe what I was telling them. They do now. *Nancy, 65, mother, Alzheimer's*

- Don't just say what a saint I am, but validate that it's a very hard job and offer to take him to the movies or something. *Marlene, 68, husband, dementia/Alzheimer's*

- I wish that I would have had the opportunity for myself and my brother to talk with someone our own age coping with something similar to us. *Andrew, 25, father, frontal lobe dementia, diagnosed at age 51*

- I wish my brother had given me more time, and when he came, it was often late in the day. *Sally, 57, mother, Alzheimer's, died 3 years after diagnosed*

- I wish I had an ethical decisions discussion with clergy. *Sandy, 61, husband, Alzheimer's and vascular dementia*

▸ Mom wishes some of the other older men in our church would have come alongside Dad and taken him on outings with them, simple stuff, out for coffee, walks, drives. *Mary, 38, father, Alzheimer's, diagnosed at age 66*

▸ Not expecting things of my husband that he can't do. *Catherine, 85, husband, Alzheimer's and Lewy Body*

▸ I would have liked my brothers to be more supportive. I had to beg some to help. Others refused, made excuses. Others I did not trust their judgment in caring for my mom so I couldn't have them help anymore. I had to put Mom's needs first. *MM, 46, mother, Alzheimer's, died 5 years after diagnosed*

213

Things I need to hear

🖉 _____

_____

_____

Things I need done

🖉 _____

_____

_____

_____

Support groups: Sharing the "nitty-gritty" of caregiving

Here's one straightforward definition of a support group:

"Your family means well. Your friends mean well. They love you. But you've got to find somebody who knows the nitty-gritty of what you're going through. The only people who know the nitty-gritty are the ones going through the same thing. You 'feed' off each other."

Another caregiver found a "wonderful" online group. The members have often been her lifeline because "nothing is off limits," including some personal topics she didn't feel comfortable sharing with her adult children …

Char didn't have the time to attend as many support group meetings as she wanted to at the very time she needed them because she was tending to the needs of her mother-in-law and mother, both diagnosed with Alzheimer's.

Oh, and those other things called everyday life, being a wife and mother, and her full-time teaching job took up most of those remaining hours. When she could attend support group sessions and caregiver seminars at the Alzheimer's Association, she found them to be very beneficial experiences.

"When you're in that room and see all these other people, it was good to connect with some of them. It helps you figure out where your person is …"

In caring for her mother, Sue has discovered that meeting other Alzheimer's families is like creating an extended family of sorts, where's she found caregivers who have become surrogate mothers. She enjoys their company because of what they have in common and are willing to share.

She applauded the local Alzheimer's Association, its caregiver workshops and huge library as a resource. Asked to join the board several years earlier, she didn't fully comprehend its offerings until faced with this role as a caregiver herself. It's there to help.

She's also been warmly greeted by the local center on aging.

"You have needs and stresses and other things going on. To have somebody ask, 'How are *you* today?' or 'How's your mom?' is very helpful because the caregivers are the ones who are really suffering. The patients don't realize it. My mom knows, but she doesn't really know ..."

Peg had a great support group, her children, as she coped with her husband's early-onset Alzheimer's.

"I had my kids, and anything I said was fine. We had friends who have been very supportive. The worse part is that when he was with me, I didn't have time to go to the support groups. I couldn't spend as much time with my friends as I wanted, but I could 'unload' on them, which definitely helped. I didn't handle it really well, but I don't know what I would have done differently."

215

However, she wasn't aware of more formal support groups in those early years. Peg can't remember who gave her the toll-free Alzheimer's Association number. She initially had to work up the courage to call but started contacting staff and volunteers often because of the positive and valuable assistance she received.

"They were so sympathetic."

For example, she recalls how her husband reacted when he saw his reflection in the mirror but didn't comprehend it was his own image. Initially thinking it was another person, he just talked. However, later, he thought there were intruders in the house, which agitated him. Peg called the 800 number, and the Alzheimer's associates suggested she put a towel over the mirror, which helped sometimes.

"They let me talk," which is what she needed most. One time, they called back the next morning with another idea to meet her immediate needs. "I was very impressed with that."

Several months after Peg placed her husband in the nursing home, she joined some support groups because she wanted to help others. "I hope I've done some good. It's therapy for me." Her friends rallied for her. "I could say anything." It does her good to talk about it, which is part of her personality. Not everybody feels comfortable doing that.

She's found many benefits from interacting with other families, no matter in what stage their loved one may be. Families welcome input, without being told what to do. They need to make their own decisions.

"They're going through enough. You try to be tactful. Each person you talk to, you play it by ear. You hope you do a little bit of good."

A letter to family & friends...

Here's how YOU can help ME cope
& survive my role as a caregiver

_____

_____

_____

_____

_____

_____

_____

_____

_____

_____

_____

_____

How will they respond?

The tough tide of transitions

"My decision was to take care of her at home. The nurse who came to our home said I was a stressed caregiver and we should make other arrangements. I'm not proud of putting her in a nursing home." Robert, 79, wife, Alzheimer's, died 6 years after diagnosed

Caregivers say...

Change is part of life, but individuals with Alzheimer's, dementia or memory loss often experience more dramatic changes that can startle or affect us deeply. It's not easy to witness.

218

What are/were the most difficult changes, both physical and emotional, exhibited by this diagnosed person that you witnessed and had to adjust to?

▶ Lost emotion

▶ Doesn't get jokes

▶ Stopping him from driving

▶ Excessive weight loss

▶ Confusion

▶ Could not recognize home of nearly 50 years

▶ Didn't clean home

▶ Didn't wash clothes

▶ Loss of ability to reason and make logical choices

▶ Constant need to go to the bathroom

▶ Fragility

▶ Age regression

▶ Anger at me

▶ Crying spells

▶ Forgetfulness

▶ Paranoia

▶ Forgetting to bathe

▶ Wandering

▶ Nocturnal snacking

▶ Restlessness

▶ No conversation

▶ Can't talk understandably

▶ Anger

▶ Destructiveness

▶ Bed wetting

▶ Coldness

▶ Losing things

▶ Verbal abuse

▶ Doesn't show or respond to affection

▶ Change of appearance

▶ Inability to walk easily

▶ Not recognizing us

▶ Loss of independence

▶ I became the parent and my mother became the child

▶ Watching her mind fade though her body was healthy

▶ The loss of their independence and ability to express themselves and of a person whose knowledge and wisdom is no longer there to reach for me as a daughter. *Christl, 55, father, stroke and Alzheimer's*

▶ Wandering off, getting lost, attitude changes, 40-50 phone calls a day because Grandma wanted to leave. *Shallen, 25, grandmother, Alzheimer's*

▶ Why she is living with us and what happened to her husband, her home, etc. *John, 67, mother-in-law, Alzheimer's*

▶ Not being able to care for herself and having to wear Depends, having many accidents. Having angry outbursts. *Jolene, 66, mother, dementia, died 5 years after diagnosed*

▶ When he started drooling and could no longer manage his secretions. It made him look so much worse in baggy, dirty clothes. *Ann, 49, mother, vascular dementia, died; father, Alzheimer's, died*

▶ I felt like I needed to charge right in there and relieve all her worries and make her feel safe. *Jenny, 56, mother, Alzheimer's*

▶ Losing all short-term memory, some angry moments. Hard to see someone once so vibrant so lost. *Mary Ann, 62, father, Alzheimer's*

▶ The blank eyes, the sparkle was gone. A once-strong lady, meek and mild, childlike. *Gayle, 59, mother, Alzheimer's, died 5 years after diagnosed*

▶ He's always cleaning out drawers, garage shelves and leaving more of a mess afterward. Not throwing anything away. *Maxine, 77, husband, Alzheimer's*

▶ It upset his life-long self-confidence. He was glad to be alive, but sad for all his lost abilities and pleasures. *Marcy, 76, husband, memory loss due to massive stroke*

"Mostly physical deterioration, 'losing' my name and lack of recognition." *Ann, 63, aunt, Alzheimer's, died 6 years after diagnosed*

▸ He became paranoid with me and other men. He said some very hurtful things. We were married more than 50 years. *Roseann, 72, husband, dementia, died 10 years after diagnosed*

▸ When she not longer could feed herself. Food had to be mashed. She could not get herself ready for bed or get dressed. *Robert, 79, wife, Alzheimer's, died 6 years after diagnosed*

▸ Not being able to do anything or understand. *David, 69, wife, Alzheimer's*

▸ Physically, he became more fragile and needed more help. Emotionally, he became less able to use good judgment, less able to accept that. *Marcy, 76, father, Alzheimer's, died 5 years after diagnosed*

▸ The slow loss of memory, physical functions and just existing. *Shirley, 72, husband, dementia*

▸ She became unable to take care of daily hygiene, didn't bathe or shower, false teeth were dirty, clothing was not kept clean. *Judith, 61, mother, Alzheimer's*

▸ The hardest is the night wandering and sometimes hurtful or inappropriate things she says. *Elizabeth, 47, mother, Alzheimer's*

▸ He frequently talked of visiting or calling his mother, who had died 17 years ago. He wanted to go "home" to his boyhood home. *Helen, 72, husband, Alzheimer's*

▸ The wasting away of his mind and body daily. Too painful for me. *Sandy, 61, husband, Alzheimer's and vascular dementia*

▸ Physically, you could start to see the life escape him when you looked in his eyes, like a shell. Emotionally for me, it was simply his initial lack of emotion or understanding. *Andrew, 25, father, frontal lobe dementia, diagnosed at age 51*

"Seeing the empty eyes. Introducing me as her sister or her mother." Elaine, 54, mother, Alzheimer's

▸ Lack of bathing, out-of-control behavior, bouncing off the walls. Gave her rags to fold one day until we got her on medication. *J, grandmother, Alzheimer's*

▸ When at sundown she forgot who I was, at first questioned me, then feared me. *Bill, 78, wife, Alzheimer's, died 4 years after diagnosed*

▸ She got to where the daily activities had to be done by me, dressing, feeding, bathing, walking with assistance near the end. Cried for no reason sometimes. Mean to my son for no reason. Wandering, not able to sit for any length of time. *MM, 46, mother, Alzheimer's, died 5 years after diagnosed*

▸ That she frequently didn't know I was her daughter and would shake her finger at me and say, "When Anne comes …" things would be better. *Anne, 67, mother, dementia, died 4 years after diagnosed*

▸ Being the dominant decision maker. Most of the time I include him in decision making. *Norma, 81, husband, Alzheimer's*

▸ Not remembering after five minutes, enhanced bad moods, argumentative behavior, acting childlike, regression. *Brian, 47, mother, Alzheimer's*

▸ One of the biggest changes is in the language. My husband was always a gentleman. He never used foul language around the house, or much at all. Suddenly it became "---- that," or "leave me the ---- alone" or "get the ---- out of here." I, who would never have used those words either, began using them back, like "One of these days you might just get what the ---- you're asking." I realize intellectually it is just frustration and that I shouldn't take it personally, but I do it anyway. When it began to be too much and my own health began to suffer, I found a day care program. *Marlene, 68, husband, dementia/Alzheimer's*

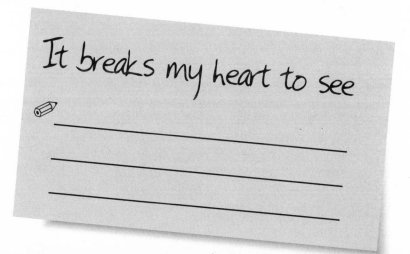

It breaks my heart to see

A matter of survival

Sometimes caregivers have to make tough decisions for the safety of the individual with dementia or memory loss and as a matter of survival for themselves.

Peg sighs as she recalls the dramatic personality changes in her husband in the fourth year after he was diagnosed with early-onset Alzheimer's. She wasn't prepared for his sudden violent behavior, horrible hallucinations and how he treated her roughly. He declined rapidly, and she had the emotional and physical challenge of evolving from the role of spouse to caregiver.

How did she cope? Their three children had been very supportive, and a neighbor "could do wonders with him when I couldn't."

"I'll be the first to admit that I didn't handle it well. I don't have a lot of patience. I tried a lot of things. I lied, I conned … that part I could handle. But when the violence started, that got very, very tough."

A few years earlier, she had an unexpected glimpse into the future. She realized about two years after his diagnosis that he didn't know her. He backhanded her if she came up behind him.

"You'd think I'd learn." She sighs.

One morning after he had hit her, she had black and blue marks on her leg. During a lucid moment, he was aghast at her bruises, having no idea he was the cause.

In the fourth year, the night heightened his violent behavior and her fears. Peg says he seemed fine the first two hours after he fell asleep, but after that, she never knew what he would do next.

One summer night he took off out the back door. She had to keep her car locked and hide the keys, By the time she got to the car, he was already two blocks away at 4 a.m. She found him talking to someone who was out walking. She explained it was a case of Alzheimer's, and that gentleman was very kind in helping her get him in her car to take him home.

The neurologist had given her medication to keep him under control during difficult periods, but Peg admits that she resisted that step for more than a year. Finally she had to administer him small doses in the final three months he was home.

"It was terrible. It was really terrible. I wouldn't wish it on my worst enemy." She believes he was mostly mad at her, though other simple things sparked his ire. For example, she turned on music, and he thought somebody was in the house trying to rob them. "Of course, it was mostly directed at me because I was the one who was there. I cried a lot."

A difficult decision could no longer be avoided.

Friends took him out to lunch every weekday for a while as she and her son used that time to research nursing homes. Only two would consider taking him because of his violent behavior.

She was home with him alone one day, and she can't even remember the specific event that "broke" her. She had finally selected a nursing facility, and on this particularly tough day, the center had an opening,

"I didn't even tell my kids until after. It was one of those things." After lunch, she took him. He became stubborn, and she filled out the papers because she couldn't take it anymore. Asked if she wanted to wait to leave until after he had settled in, she declined. She was emotionally and physically exhausted.

"I was scared, I think. I just left. I actually hated him. It really bothered me when I took him to the nursing home. Thank goodness the feeling only lasted a few days. I guess I was having selfish thoughts, 'Why was I going through this?' When you're going through it, you don't have time to think. That was very tough. I think it was tougher on the kids than me. They watched as it progressed. I hid a lot from the kids. I don't know why I did. I thought they wouldn't have to go through it if they didn't know."

She has no regrets for her difficult, though necessary, decision.

"You just live every day for what it is."

What's my breaking point?

_____

_____

_____

Professionals say...

Dementia and memory loss patients are not immune to having just an ordinary bad day like the rest of us.

224 **What advice do you have for families when the patient has a bad day?**

▶ Don't take it personal because the next visit they won't even remember. *Latoya, 27, CNA, 2 years*

▶ That this is not a normal day for them, that staff will help ease their concern/problem. *Kalah, 48, social service assistant, four months*

▶ Come back another day. *Pam, 44, LPN, 25 years*

▶ Everyone has a bad day. *Dave, 40, executive director, 2 years*

▶ Let them rest, get them out of over-stimulating environments. Soft music is great. *Cindy, 53, nurse, 34 years*

▶ Just spend quiet time together. *Marge, 50, nursing home administrator, 24 years*

▶ Try to put yourself in their place. *Sherry, 27, trainer, 2 years*

▶ Allow others to intervene with respite. *Ronni, R.N, 49, 28 years*

▶ Tomorrow will be different. *Sharon, 55, nurse aide/driver, 15 years*

▶ Be understanding. Try to give them feel a reason to be positive. *Michelle, 48, CNA, 30 years*

▶ Try and remember something that was fun or good. Remember they are not going to remember what is going on five minutes later. *Gloria, 54, CNA, 18 years*

▶ Bear with them. Try to understand. Remember the person as they once were and remember the love for that person. *Karen, 46, developmental technician, 20 years*

▶ Talk to the patient. Let them know we sometimes have bad days. *Debi, 48, trainer, 6 years*

▶ Everyone has a bad day. Start tomorrow and treat it as a new day. *Mary, 37, hospital social worker, 11 years*

- Listen, use life stories. *Edi, social worker, 17 years*

- Sit with them, hold their hand if they like it, walk. *Trudy, 57, director of nursing, 30 years*

- It won't always be bad. We all have had bad days. Think of the good days. They are not really blaming you. *Vicki, 56, R.N., 35 years*

- Back off. *Susan, 58, LPN*

225

One way to stop a "thief"

You go and visit someone with dementia or memory loss, and after you leave, that individual accuses *you* of stealing her purse because "it's gone!"

Many individuals with dementia or memory loss often believe that someone is stealing from them because they can't find the items they've innocently misplaced themselves.

Before she joined the Alzheimer's Association as a patient and family services coordinator, Alisha worked in an assisted living facility and came across numerous incidents of "thievery."

"Their brains are making up stuff to deal with and make sense of their world. They still have emotions," she explains. Sometimes they'll demand someone call the police and report this "robbery."

She remembers one woman who was so insistent on calling the police herself that the staff rigged a call, dialing a number so that this woman thought she was talking to the police.

"She feels better that she's talking to the authorities, and her day is better for that. To me, that's not lying; that is living in her world."

Find what works to acknowledge their emotions and role play if necessary. While the staff obviously wouldn't bother the police with this matter, this small effort gave her peace of mind.

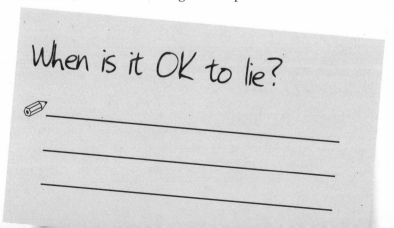

When is it OK to lie?

Caregivers say...

What saddened you the most?

226

- Loss of memory
- Not knowing me or my name
- Unable to multi-task
- When he became incontinent
- Loss of independence
- Losing the will to live
- His vulnerability
- Loss of her advice
- The empty stare
- Losing my mother to the disease
- Watching her struggle

- Witnessing her fear
- Not knowing what food he likes
- Inability to travel anymore
- His sadness over the loss of his intelligence
- Watching her memory slip away slowly
- The confusion
- Unable to speak
- Unable to read
- Unable to interact
- She couldn't say "I love you" anymore

- Knowing what is coming next. *Laurie, 47, father, dementia*
- When she talks about her deceased husband as being alive. *John, 67, mother-in-law, Alzheimer's*
- When he couldn't hug me back. *Ann, 49, mother, vascular dementia, died; father, Alzheimer's, died*

"Watching a man with a Ph.D not be able to find his way home!" Helen, 72, husband, Alzheimer's

- I've lost my husband, but he's still here. *Pat, 66, husband, Alzheimer's*
- To watch him progress rapidly to severe stages. *Mary Ann, 62, father, Alzheimer's*
- Putting him in the home was worse than his death. *Edna, 83, husband, Alzheimer's, died 7 years after diagnosed*

- When she asked me if I could find her husband for her. *Robert, 79, wife, Alzheimer's, died 6 years after diagnosed*

- Loss of the essence. *Ann, 63, aunt, Alzheimer's, died 6 years after diagnosed*

- Loss of friends and relatives. *David, 69, wife, Alzheimer's*

- To see his feelings of helplessness, of necessary dependence. *Marcy, 76, father, Alzheimer's, died 5 years after diagnosed*

227

- When she was aware of her confusion, seeing her frustration. *Judith, 61, mother, Alzheimer's*

- She felt I wasn't there for her. *Anne, 67, mother, dementia, died 4 years after diagnosed*

- Her pleading, begging, crying. *Elaine, 54, mother, Alzheimer's*

- Her lack of remembering anything of life in later years. *Nancy, 65, mother, Alzheimer's*

- That we both lost years of a healthy shared retirement. *Marcy, 76, husband, memory loss due to massive stroke*

- The confusion. I can't call her and talk for hours like in the old days. *Kevin, 45, mother, Alzheimer's*

- The thought of my mom and how she would cope. *Andrew, 25, father, frontal lobe dementia, diagnosed at age 51*

- That she forgot who I was after 50 years. *Bill, 78, wife, Alzheimer's, died 4 years after diagnosed*

- Losing my daddy. He's still a decent man, but not my Dad. His stupid jokes and sense of humor are gone. *Mary, 38, father, Alzheimer's*

- Mom believed that her children were against her, after her money and possessions. *Jody, 47, mother, early onset Alzheimer's*

- When I thought of the future, what it could be like. *Norma, 81, husband, Alzheimer's*

"When he said to me, 'I'm doing the best I can.'" *Leora, 72, husband, Alzheimer's*

"She thought I was stealing things, that I was the bad guy"

Coping with a loved one's memory loss would be enough for one family, but Char and Jim have had to face it a second time.

How this couple dealt with Jim's mother's Alzheimer's is recounted earlier in this volume. Here's how they've addressed the same diagnosis in Char's mother.

As a widow, this woman continued to enjoy life and participate in a variety of activities. Though she was still quite vibrant at age 80, Char and Jim began to notice her taking on some different personality traits, specifically a growing sense of paranoia and a lot of anger. Char kept meticulous notes to share with her mother's physician to make it easy for him.

Suddenly, a great deal of her indignation targeted her daughter, with whom she had always gotten along well. Jim and Char painted her house of a half-century and because of the movement of items, she accused Char of stealing.

"Okay," Jim says, "we're thinking that she doesn't have a handle on things like we thought she did." Char's mom thought there were two Chars, the good one and the bad one, and referred to the bad one as that "other woman." "I was in her good graces. She'd say, 'I trust you (Jim), but that other woman is robbing me blind.' "

Char remembers how her paranoia escalated as she changed the house locks and started hiding her purse. Over time, she had called every locksmith in town.

"She thought I was stealing things, that I was the bad guy. I was the extremely horrible daughter."

Jim says she started telling friends and neighbors that Char was stealing stuff. It wasn't long before these people began to wonder what was wrong with the mother, who told Jim how terrible his wife was. He often wonders if she asked herself why she can't remember things.

"You can't keep track of everything."

Jim concurs. It's hard enough to take care of yourself and keep track of everything, but "you have to be their brain, too. We're the ones who had to implement things and make them work. She'd never have answers to logical questions. But you had to deal with their anger and confusion because it didn't go away."

They could not ignore other changes over time. She'd forget to put something back in the refrigerator. She was unable to hang up a phone. She couldn't follow the steps to use the microwave. She could read but couldn't comprehend the words. She couldn't even state her age. One day Jim searched everywhere for his eyeglasses and discovered his mother-in-law was wearing them.

It's a disease that people have trouble accepting, he adds. There's no getting better, and it defies logic. Her mom would talk and make no sense. She confused the phone and remote. He recalls telling her on the phone how to jiggle the toilet handle because the water was running continuously.

They decided to move her into an assisted living facility.

"We took care of her house and yard for 10 years. She said, 'Why should I move? I like it here.' " Disease or not, Jim finally lost his patience with her. " 'Yeah, you do nothing. It's like living in a hotel. You don't cook, you don't clean. We're doing all this for 10 years. We're getting tired of spending every weekend here.' "

"Working with little kids," Char says, "was a diversion. While I'm at school teaching first graders, I'm not thinking about her every minute. At one point, I was so frustrated with my mother's behavior that I wrote her a letter because I couldn't talk to her. She wouldn't hear me. I'd cry on my way home after Mom was nasty to me. She was always angry at me."

Though the daughter admits she felt guilt initially placing her in assisted living, "everything's fine in her own little world," Char says. At least they're not worried now about her letting strangers into her home.

Char still checks on her several times a week because they have to monitor how she's doing and make sure that medications are being administered properly and that others are not being prescribed without family approval.

Consider these observations:

▸ *Years of habits allowed Char's mother to continue certain routines.*

▸ *Some big expenses were found to be purchases of duplicate items because her mother couldn't remember she already had the items.*

▸ *She was good at masking difficulties for a long time.*

▶ *Plan ahead and get the individual's name on a list at your preferred healthcare facility.*

▶ *"Sometimes they give you the answer you want because they don't want to be questioned."*

▶ *You have to be forceful with them at times. "Sit there until I get back." They follow anyway.*

▶ *"In Alzheimer's, there's nothing to come back to."*

"You can't rationalize with an Alzheimer's patient," Jim adds. "That's hard to get across. Some things come up that go against human logic. You can't take a pill. You can't run to the doctor."

Here are excerpts from Char's letter to her mother, written out of the frustration she experienced in response to her mother's accusations of stealing.

Your home was in total chaos while the painting and carpeting was getting done ... You insisted on putting things back by yourself as you said you wanted to clean out drawers and cabinets. This was an overwhelming task. You were always looking for something. Nearly daily you called me if I had seen a missing article. When you couldn't find what you were looking for, your frustration became more and more evident and that's when the accusations began. You seemed to be transferring that exasperation to me in the form of blame. Since that time you have accused me of taking many things that I had no reason or need to take ... The situation has gotten worse in the past year. Perhaps the possibility exists that you don't remember where you put things. We all misplace items from time to time. You also have been known to hide things in closets, drawers or under tablecloths, etc.

It seems you lose things often — maybe more than most people. As we age, our brains just don't recall details as easily — details like where you have put something. Accept this fact and deal with it. One thing is certain. I have never stolen anything from you or out of your house. I have not borrowed anything and not returned it. I am afraid to borrow something for fear you won't remember I returned it! I resent this continual abuse and am asking you to stop leaving notes telling me not to steal. I do honor the commandment give by God —"Thou shall not steal."

If you want any kind of mother/daughter relationship at all, you need to come to terms with these issues. It seems so unhealthy to let this problem continue without trying to resolve it. I love you dearly and do not want these issues to drive a wedge between you and me or my family.

A letter to my loved one...

Dear

I want to tell you how I feel

_____

_____

_____

_____

_____

_____

_____

_____

_____

_____

_____

How would they respond?

Role changes require patience, understanding

With dementia and memory loss, family members often find themselves having to adjust to new roles.

Bonnie, education specialist at the Alzheimer's Association, says spouses often assume new gender roles in relationships.

"We've got men who need to figure out how to cook, clean, go buy bras, whatever, that they've never done. And we have women who've never written a check, dealt with insurance and finances. They're losing and adding roles and responsibilities that people are not necessarily prepared for because they don't expect that to happen ..."

"One of the biggest challenges has been the role reversal," says Sue. "They're not ... Oh, I'll probably cry now ... They're not your mom anymore. They're imprisoned in their bodies. My mother was a very strong person, volunteered everywhere, gave, gave, gave to the community. Fully in charge of the household ... to see her not able to make a decision or write a check ... to depend on you for everything is very hard to watch ..."

Norma writes that "in the case of a parent, you must get used to switching roles with them. They are no longer the person you relied on for answers. You are now the one in charge ..."

Elizabeth says, "It also meant a complete change in our relationship, like giving her a shower or wiping her bottom ..."

Pam learned a great deal about her father's past during his Alzheimer's. The era that locked him in the tightest was World War II. At one point, to engage this military sergeant in any conversation, she pretended to be his former captain. He relived experiences, such as saving a doll to give a girl being evacuated during the war.

When living with her, he wanted ice cream at 4 a.m. one morning. He didn't need drugs; he needed a hot fudge sundae. At one point, he refused to ride with her until she donned a chauffeur's cap.

Once as she ran errands, he locked himself in her car. She finally had to call emergency personnel. When they called him

"Sergeant," he agreed to emerge. They had to communicate with him at the place where he was in his mind.

"You do what you've got to do," Pam adds ...

How did one woman adapt to changing her role from wife to caregiver?

"Not easily. Because I knew I had to, I knew I didn't have a choice. I had to separate the two because it was breaking my heart too much. I had to convince myself to take two steps away to become the caregiver. I had to realize that our days together as husband and wife, as lovers were over.

"It was hard, very difficult for both of us. He lost the mechanics of making love. He couldn't remember how, and it got to be too frustrating for both of us, and we'd end up in tears. I finally said, 'You know, we don't need that anyway.' I just made a joke of it. 'Let's just snuggle.' That was okay."

He started jerking during the night and unintentionally slugged her, leaving nasty bruises. She finally had to move into another bedroom.

"Someone's going to think I'm a battered wife. That was one of the most difficult things to accept that we weren't going to have that part of our lives."

Then it became easier to care for him. It was the only way she could cope by severing some of the emotional ties.

"I don't know how people do it otherwise, but everybody's different. I couldn't be both to him. I had to be his caregiver and give up the other part."

233

How am I adapting?

_____

_____

_____

_____

_____

_____

Caregivers say...

Many, if not most, families of dementia and memory loss clients face the difficult decision of placing their loved one in a long-term care facility because the health and well-being of the individual and perhaps even the immediate caregiver is now in jeopardy. Each family must make those decisions based on its unique needs and circumstances.

How were decisions made concerning the long-term care of this person, whether they remained at home or were placed in a nursing home/facility?

▶ Individual, family and physician discussed it

▶ Hired a long-term caregiver to keep him in his home

▶ Family concurred

▶ Made decision based on doctor's advice

▶ Selected nursing home with Alzheimer's unit

▶ Placed her in a nursing home when she needed pureed foods

▶ Lots of open discussion and research

▶ Interviewed and visited nursing homes early enough to not be rushed into a decision

▶ Primary caregiver made decisions and sought siblings' input

▶ Sent family members to Alzheimer's Association for education

▶ It became too hard to deal with, so they chose to put her in a home for 24-hour care. *Shallen, 25, grandmother, Alzheimer's*

▶ The family decided to wait until safety is an issue or incontinence before nursing facility placement. *Laurie, 47, father, dementia*

▶ Forced in part. They were living in an assisted living facility that really wasn't set up the way they promoted themselves. The level of assistance didn't match the need. *Ann, 49, mother, vascular dementia, died; father, Alzheimer's, died*

▸ We asked her, and so far she is doing fine. We take her on vacation to Florida for the winter, and she is active in clubhouse activities. *John, 67, mother-in-law, Alzheimer's*

▸ Social service department made arrangements for the nursing home. I wasn't strong enough for one caregiver. *Jolene, 66, mother, dementia, died 5 years after diagnosed*

▸ I had discussed it with the children. I just didn't know when. *Edna, 83, husband, Alzheimer's, died 7 years after diagnosed*

235

▸ Our daughter encouraged me to plan for it, especially in case I would become sick. She lived out of town. *Leora, 72, husband, Alzheimer's*

▸ For my mother, her husband was in charge and even when I went to a lawyer to try to take her to a nursing home, they wouldn't let me. *Norma, 81, mother, Alzheimer's, died 11 years after diagnosed; sister, Alzheimer's, died 6 years after diagnosed*

▸ I am a nurse, and I would not wish a nursing home and/or hospital on someone with memory problems without family there daily to oversee their care. *Nettie, 51, father, Alzheimer's*

▸ She chose the group home. When they could no longer keep her, I moved her to an Alzheimer's facility near my home. *Ann, 63, aunt, Alzheimer's, died 6 years after diagnosed*

▸ My children will insist on nursing home care when they feel it's needed. *Helen, 72, husband, Alzheimer's*

▸ When I couldn't manage his condition after falling, his doctor arranged for his placement in a nursing home. *Marcy, 76, father, Alzheimer's, died 5 years after diagnosed*

▸ He was in the hospital, and I could no longer care for him because he kept falling and I couldn't get him up. *Shirley, 72, husband, dementia*

"When Dad could no longer take care of her, I was told I had to take her. When I couldn't handle her anymore, I made the decision to put her in the nursing home." *Darlene, 58, mother, Alzheimer's*

▶ Easily. We had few choices. *Nancy, 65, mother, Alzheimer's*

▶ He is currently at home. There are times when I think I can't do this any longer. Luckily, financially we are able to hire companions. I don't know how people without much money can manage. I know they do. They have to, and my heart hurts for all of us, the affected and caregivers. This is a terrible, terrible disease. *Marlene, 68, husband, dementia/Alzheimer's*

▶ He's at home as long as I can care for him. If I can no longer do that, he will be placed in a Medicaid facility. Not much choice. *Marcy, 76, husband, memory loss due to massive stroke*

▶ We decided that as soon as he gave us a sign — did something outrageous — we would know it was time. We prayed for that sign, to be strong enough to know, but not too strong, of course. *Andrew, 25, father, frontal lobe dementia, diagnosed at age 51*

▶ My husband and I decided that as long as she knew us, she remained at home. *Sally, 57, mother, Alzheimer's, died 3 years after diagnosed*

▶ Money! If he goes into a nursing home, I have to go back to work to pay for it. Who would want a RN at my age? *Sandy, 61, husband, Alzheimer's and vascular dementia*

▶ Our four children realized they were losing their mother and didn't want to lose their father, too. *Bill, 78, wife, Alzheimer's, died 4 years after diagnosed*

"I told him I would care for him at home as long as I could, then a care center. When that time came, we started looking together, found one and he settled in pretty well." Roseann, 72, husband, dementia, died 10 years after diagnosed

▶ She was in the hospital two different times, and the last time the doctor would not let me take her home. I was unable to take care of her. *MM, 46, mother, Alzheimer's, died 5 years after diagnosed*

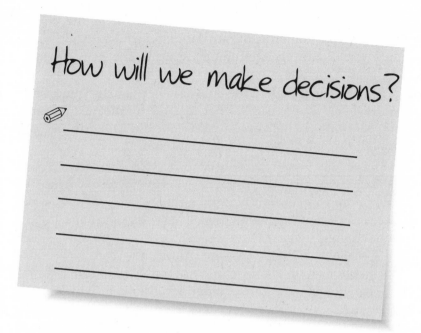

How will we make decisions?

After 61 years of marriage, I am still dating my wife

From Tom

At the bus station in December 1944, I spotted this beautiful auburn-haired girl. The good Lord was with me as they announced that all buses were canceled because of the ice storm. I seized the opportunity and offered to help this beautiful young lady and her sister carry their luggage to the train station. We visited on the ride, and I found out that she only lived a short distance from me and that we both used the same local bus.

This beautiful girl, Laura, consented to dating me. From that moment on, I never dated or even looked at another girl. In fall 1945, I decided to ask her to marry me. We planned to go out to dinner, and I wanted to make it a special time. I bought a corsage and had the florist neatly tie the engagement ring into the corsage and place it in a fancy white box. When she opened the box, I asked her to marry me. She said yes, and in December, we held hands as walked down the aisle to say our wedding vows.

Our first wedding anniversary was spent in the delivery room awaiting the birth of our daughter, who arrived the next day. We really appreciated this blessing as she grew up so fast and had a daughter of her own.

In 1996, Laura suffered what was believed to be some kind of seizure. I was able to care for her at home for the next five and a half years with the help of our doctor, the day care unit and guidance of the local Alzheimer's support group.

These years were more tiring than I ever realized at the time. Laura was constantly putting things away for safekeeping and then not remembering where she put them. I had to remind myself time and time again that Laura was not to blame, that Alzheimer's disease was the culprit.

I had to lock up all medicines or Laura would think the pills were candy and start eating them. I had to deal with personal issues such as cleanliness, brushing teeth, combing hair, bathing, etc. I had to install security systems on stairs, cabinets, drawers and doors to keep her from getting hurt. I had to help her select and then put on suitable clothes for weather conditions.

Interesting item here. Men, have you ever attempted to find suitable underwear for your wife when size labels on existing clothes either been removed or faded? I was rescued by a lady sales clerk.

Eating is another major problem. You try to guess what they will eat at a given time. This becomes a special problem when you are at a restaurant and you are trying to describe what is on the menu.

Laura and many others with Alzheimer's are unable to make decisions, and if you make a decision for them and it turns out to be the wrong one, then you are in trouble. It may take a while to get things straightened out without losing your temper.

Other situations included walking away from me in a store, picking up items believing they belonged to her and incontinence when out in public. One time, Laura was in the early stages and needed to go to the bathroom at a restaurant. I took her to the door of the ladies' restroom. She went in but did not come out. After waiting for a short time, I asked a waitress to go in and check on her. The door had an automatic lock mechanism on it for privacy and you had to turn a special button on the knob to open the door from the inside. Try to explain this to a terrified Alzheimer's patient. We finally had to have a manager unlock the door. Total time: nearly a hour.

Even though adult day care relieved me of some of these problems, I still had to get her up in the morning, get her dressed, feed her and take her to day care. I still faced these problems as soon as she came home. Day care did give me time to accomplish things that I could not do when Laura was home and needed my full attention.

239

The hardest day of my life was when I took Laura to the nursing home. While I was taking care of paperwork, one of the aides came over, introduced herself to Laura, took her by the hand and said, "let me show you around." I think Laura's experience at the day care paid off as she got up and away they went.

When I left after signing the paperwork, I had tears thinking that I was no longer able to take care of my beautiful wife. When I came back that afternoon to visit, she was in the lounge with some of the residents watching TV or doing something else. I was very pleased to see how happy and contented she was.

She loves the nursing staff, and they all seem to like her. When Laura was still able to walk, the nursing staff would get her ready for me to take her for afternoon car rides. They now get her ready for me to wheel her out to the large swing. Laura loves to swing and many times she will give the nursing staff a big smile as they rub suntan lotion on her face and arms. As I push the wheelchair, many of the ladies will make very nice remarks about that beautiful girl with the cowgirl hat, and Laura will give them a big smile.

I used to visit Laura every afternoon and evening, and then one night I noticed that all of the other residents had gone to bed. I asked if they were keeping Laura up just so I could visit her. They said yes.

I appreciated this extra effort on the part of the staff and suggested they put her to bed at the same time as the others. I am now dating Laura every afternoon from 3:30 until dinner time.

Professionals say...

When a dementia or memory loss patient moves into a healthcare facility, the family's responsibility does not end there. Families are still vitally important to enhancing the patients' daily life.

How can families be included in the care process if their loved ones are in a facility?

▶ They could come in and help with activities of daily life (ADL's) or other favorite activities. *Latoya, 27, CNA, 2 years*

▶ Volunteer, participate. *Kalah, 48, social service assistant, four months*

▶ Include them in their care plans. *Pam, 44, LPN, 25 years*

▶ Visit anytime without expectations. *Dave, 40, executive director, 2 years*

▶ Establish a family environment; establish close ties. Have family-oriented activities. Keep them informed of what's going on. *Cindy, 53, nurse, 34 years*

▶ Take time to invite family and the resident to sit and chat on a regular basis. *Marge, 50, nursing home administrator, 24 years*

▶ Come in and visit the loved one, call to check on how they are doing, etc. *Sherry, 27, trainer, 2 years*

▶ Involvement in care planning, activities, visits, etc. *Ronni, R.N, 49, 28 years*

▶ Bringing in old photos or a favorite food. *Sharon, 55, nurse aide/driver, 15 years*

▶ Frequent contact. Tell them anecdotes about loved ones. *Connie, 57, psychotherapist*

▶ Constant involvement, be positive and encouraging. *Michelle, 48, CNA, 30 years*

▶ Try and go at least one time a day and make it early in the day or when they are eating. *Gloria, 54, CNA, 18 years*

▶ Attend care plan meetings. *Susan, 38, R.N., 12 years*

▸ Families' voice needs to be listened to as well. *Edi, social worker, 17 years*

▸ Be included! Don't drop them off and never go back just because "they'll never know if I'm there or not." Are you sure about that? *Karen, 46, developmental technician, 20 years*

▸ Letting them know that their family member needs to have them involved in their life. *Debi, 48, trainer, 6 years*

241

▸ Talk about their life, bring familiar things, eat with them. *Trudy, 57, director of nursing, 30 years*

▸ Include them in activities and their care. They can still take them out for things. *Vicki, 56, R.N., 35 years*

▸ Involve in care plans and ask families of residents about past times, work, pets. etc. *Susan, 58, LPN*

Questions I can ask staff

_____

_____

_____

_____

_____

_____

"Keep them engaged and going for as long as possible"

Some are engaged. Some are observers. Some will sing along with a familiar tune or tap their feet. Some walk the hallway with its safety rail. Some will say nothing for hours. Some chatter to nobody in particular.

More than half of the 100 individuals who attend this adult day care center have dementia or memory loss. About 40 attend on any weekday, giving their immediate caregivers the time to run errands, work or simply rest.

"We're giving quality of life to the caregiver," says Lori, social services coordinator. "We're giving quality of life to the participant. We reduce the stress on the caregiver so they can continue to care for them longer."

Complete with nurses on staff, and a hospital bed in a separate room to isolate anyone who becomes ill, the program features a safe, comfortable and friendly environment for adults who need some assistance and, for their own safety, should not be left alone.

The staff posts and announces the activity schedule every morning as participants trickle in for the day. Social time offers as much interaction as the client wants. Lori says that they try to keep them engaged as much as possible and do their best to honor many families' requests that they not rest too much so that they'll sleep at night at home.

There is a television, but it's not used much because clients generally have that at home, though they have the occasional movie and popcorn. Breakfast is available if desired and is followed at 10 a.m. by announcements and a short round of "sitercise" to keep them limber and awake.

"They get out of it what they put into it. Our staff walks around and encourages them to participate," she explains. They must have a doctor's authorization to exercise, and most of the time, 100 percent are eligible. If they're not, they're involved in another activity.

Morning mental stimulation activities include any topic from Bible study to trivia, a discussion about the latest news and personalities, and music to help them remember words. After lunch, they participate in other activities such as table games, and, weather permitting, go out into the lock-secured courtyard. An alarm goes off if someone goes out unattended. They practice safety procedures every month, which will hopefully help them remember in case of an emergency.

Also available are handicapped-accessible restrooms with a shower if needed, and cabinets for clothing changes. Adjacent to this center is a rehabilitation facility, which is handy for those participants who require physical or restorative therapy.

243

While this center gets funding from a variety of sources, including what a client pays, it's still far less expensive than home health care, Lori says. The environment provides valuable social interaction for the clients and provides a worry-free setting for often overworked caregivers.

"We may have clients who are impaired cognitively, but I've watched other participants take care of them. It's a family environment. If they need a glass or water or directions to the bathroom, it's good seeing them take these new friends under their wing and accepting them. It's a wonderful thing to see."

Some families and participants are wary of adding the adult day care component, but Lori says the staff has seen a positive response once they're in the door. It isn't long before they hear from families about the many benefits derived from the experience.

Caregivers can accomplish things that they couldn't before, and participants are performing simple tasks by just getting ready for the day, which they may have ignored if they were home all the time. Lori notes that many caregivers report their loved ones are even describing what they did at the center during the day. Even those who can't convey experiences verbally are often more energized. What's even better in some cases is that the client is exhausted at the end of day and sleeps better at night, which is also good for the caregiver.

Adult day care isn't for everyone at any stage. This social environment may not work for those clients who are later in the cognitive decline process. Caregivers keep saying they're going to bring them, but by the time they call this agency, it may be too late to be of any benefit, she adds.

Clients still want to feel useful and appreciated, so the staff often provides a healthy "therapeutic fib," when a client is "hired" for the day and paid with money the caregiver leaves. If it helps with the adjustment, they do it.

Lori tells of one son whose mother "volunteered" to be a typist, and that's all she did the first couple of weeks. She had to take breaks, and she'd mingle. After a while, she asked if she could play bingo or cards. Finally, she didn't want to work anymore but just enjoy herself. One gentleman was a greeter and helped push wheelchairs.

"We want to work with families to make this a positive experience," even if means telling the clients they're going to work or volunteer.

"There is something special about this program, these people. Yes, they have memory loss, but they're still there. What we want to do is bring that person out and keep them engaged and going for as long as possible." She recalls one woman who had significant cognitive impairment, but occasionally she'd say something that showed that her essence was still there. "We're giving her that stimulation to allow her to reach out to us. It's amazing to see little things like that."

244

How can I preserve dignity?

Caregiving without guilt: "Nobody is blaming you"

The powerful emotion of guilt seems ready to pounce upon caregivers the instant they question any of their decisions. For those who care for loved ones with dementia or memory loss, that guilt can be magnified when the individual can't communicate their wishes or how they feel.

That uneasiness reaches its peak when a caregiver must decide to place someone in adult day care, assisted living or a nursing home. That decision must not be clouded by guilt or a sense of failure, but a focus on what is best for the safety and health of the loved one.

"Everybody's afraid to do the wrong thing," says Bonnie, education specialist at the Alzheimer's Association. " 'What if … I take them to the nursing home and it's the not the right thing or I take them to day care?' I try to tell people that whatever you do is not set in stone. If after a while, if it's not the right thing, you can do something different. You can change your mind."

Some guilt has eased thanks to more awareness and options.

"We stress that you can't do it alone,"she explains. "And you can't do it perfectly, because there is no perfect. People with dementia are too unpredictable, and once you think it's working, it's going to change. It's just like raising a kid. That's just the way it is. You've got to be flexible."

Bonnie has encouraging news for caregivers: she's encountered many dementia and memory loss clients who, in lucid moments, have worried that their caregivers would risk their own health.

"They were afraid the caregiver would keep trying to have them at home or wherever for longer than they should or are able, to the point where it impacts their health."

Since many caregivers are in their 70s or 80s, that creates a lot of physical and emotional stress, though they try to hide it. Or they're sticking to a promise they made to never place a loved one in a nursing home, "which you should never promise anyone," she says.

Some caregivers even hesitate taking them to adult day care. By then, the person may not be communicating much anyway, but they have a close tie to their caregiver because that person gives them a sense of identity. The caregiver then decides the individual with dementia or memory loss doesn't want to go.

However, "you need the break and it's better for them," she stresses. Alzheimer's staff members have discovered over again that the clients really do enjoy going.

Sue faced those guilty emotions when she and her husband planned to go away for a weekend, and she would have someone fill in. It was her mother who asked, "You wouldn't leave me alone, would you?" Sue immediately reassured her that she would never do that.

"That was heartbreaking. They sort of know, yet they don't."

After several years of home care, Sue had to consider assisted living. As the only adult child who lived in town, she conferred with her siblings and explained why.

"I don't think they realized what I was doing here, bathing her, things like that. They all supported it with one exception, my youngest brother, who I don't think could deal with it. My sister and I proceeded anyway. He said she'd die if she went into a nursing home.

"I said, 'First of all, this isn't a nursing home. And second of all, she's going to die anyway from a fall or something in the house.' But he got so angry, he did not speak to me through the holidays. On New Year's, we managed to reconcile. It's a very hard thing on families. You suffer more than they do. In my mom's case, she was very comfortable and didn't realize where she was."

Eventually her brother came around, and she helped him ease his guilt. "Nobody is blaming you."

"I do think people need to give themselves permission that when the time comes when they can no longer do it, that it's okay. It's very hard, and you have a lot of guilt," she explains.

"I remember her first nights at the assisted living center, she looked for me day and night three solid days. It was just awful. I'd go home and say, 'I can't leave her there. I'm bringing her back.' But I stuck it out, and it was the right thing to do. It will be okay and they'll do fine. They'll make new friends, and it's a good thing for them."

Sue stresses that assisted living does not relieve a caregiver of all responsibilities.

"You have to go set up meds and watch everything. You still take them to the doctor. You just feel helpless to do everything they need, all the little things. It's not skilled care, but it's good. It was a very difficult decision to make. You feel like, 'I should be able to do this.' But then I saw that she was getting so much more in terms of activities and stimulation than I could offer. She was isolated from people her age at home. In many ways, it's good for her to be around people her age. You kind of get through that guilt in having to place them when you see that they're getting something you can't give them.

247

"Give yourself permission to do what is best without feeling guilty. I believe in my heart that if she were in her right mind, she would not want anybody to feel guilty. I know what kind of person she was. I try to make all decisions based on what I know about her, what she would like, want or do. It's the best you can do. If you can't do anymore, you can't. I've come to terms with that, I think …"

Vicky faced decision after decision and had to get past any guilt to make the safest and most economical choices for her husband Tom's personal care as they coped with his early-onset Alzheimer's.

Since he was not wandering much, she opted for adult day care a couple days a week while someone came into the home the other three weekdays. He thought the day care was his job, and she would slip money to the operator to give Tom as pay at the end of week. Then he'd give it to her to help pay bills.

"That way he was 'helping those old people' and working."

It wasn't long before his wandering got out of control, even in their own home. He would unknowingly hide around the house, and she'd have to search for him. She had to call the police a couple of times to find him when he wandered off their property.

Soon, Tom would wake up seven or eight times a night while she was trying to sleep to go to work. She couldn't afford any more help at home, and assistance from a program to keep people under age 60 out of the nursing home wasn't enough. They were losing money, and her only option was to place him in a nursing home.

"The state will pay for a person to be in a nursing home but not half that amount to help keep them at home. That was the final …"

Her voice breaks as she relives that terrible episode.

"We were broke … I had to have help … He was getting worse. I couldn't quit my job because we needed the money and the insurance, but I couldn't be up all night every night. I had alarms everywhere in the house. I knew the minute he walked out of his room. I had alarms and deadbolts, but he still managed to get out."

He may have only slept two hours, but to him, he had slept all night and was ready to go for the day.

What did their children say?

"They thought I was pushing it and rushing things. They thought it was wrong. I said, 'It's not where I want him to be, but where he needs to be.' "

She picked him up on weekends in the beginning to bring him home. Often she'd take him out to watch the grandkids play ball. In late winter, she had taken him to a granddaughter's basketball game, but he kept wandering away.

"It took me 45 minutes to get him in the car. He didn't understand the mechanics of sitting in the car. I could not get him in the car literally. I just couldn't do this anymore."

What guilt must I resolve?

Professionals say...

Individuals who work in long-term healthcare facilities witness the special and ordinary days and events that go on in their patients' lives. Just by keeping their eyes and ears open, they've learned much on how to lift everyone's day.

What family or visitor behaviors have you observed that benefited the patient?

▸ Visits where the visitor brought in a favorite pet or food of some kind that they haven't had in a while. *Latoya, 27, CNA, 2 years*

▸ Openness, acceptance of residents' health change, patience. *Kalah, 48, social service assistant, four months*

▸ Going with the flow and having patience. Don't totally interrupt the moment. *Dave, 40, executive director, 2 years*

▸ One-on-one stimulation. *Cindy, 53, nurse, 34 years*

▸ Touching, hugging is very powerful. *Marge, 50, nursing home administrator, 24 years*

▸ Being nice and understanding. *Sherry, 27, trainer, 2 years*

▸ Caring, calm and gentle mannerisms. *Ronni, R.N, 49, 28 years*

▸ Reminiscing about the past and bringing in the family dog. *Sharon, 55, nurse aide/driver, 15 years*

▸ Bringing pictures to look at. Doing manicures or facials. *Susan, 38, R.N., 12 years*

▸ Children. They always seem to put a sparkle in their eyes. *Karen, 46, developmental technician, 20 years*

▸ Let the patient choose the topic of conversation and lead it. *Mary, 37, hospital social worker, 11 years*

▸ Adapt to where they are in the disease. *Trudy, 57, director of nursing, 30 years*

▸ Just talking, instead of questioning. *Debi, 48, trainer, 6 years*

▸ Smiling and spending time with them, doing things, activities, etc. with them. *Vicki, 56, R.N., 35 years*

▸ Religion. *Susan, 58, LPN*

What activities can families or visitors do to make visits more enjoyable for everyone?

▸ Any activities that they enjoyed doing as a family before the disease developed. *Latoya, 27, CNA, 2 years*

▸ Participate in organized programs. Volunteer. *Kalah, 48, social service assistant, four months*

▸ Relax and follow the resident's lead. Join in whatever is going on. *Dave, 40, executive director, 2 years*

▸ Reminisce, sing. They love to play catch with a large, safe ball. *Cindy, 53, nurse, 34 years*

▸ Seek out a quiet area to visit in. *Marge, 50, nursing home administrator, 24 years*

▸ Allow staff insight into patient's likes, dislikes, and history, social, family, behavioral. *Ronni, R.N, 49, 28 years*

▸ Do something that makes the patient smile. *Sharon, 55, nurse aide/driver, 15 years*

▸ Show respect, go outside, go out to eat, hug, say "I love you." *Connie, 57, psychotherapist*

▸ Visit often. Make patients or family members feel valued. *Michelle, 48, CNA, 30 years*

▸ Bring pictures that incorporate what they do remember into what they have forgotten. *Karen, 46, developmental technician, 20 years*

▸ Games, talking about recipes they might like, bringing familiar items from home. *Debi, 48, trainer, 6 years*

▸ Activities that they all did before and enjoyed, something that includes their life story. *Vicki, 56, R.N., 35 years*

▸ Apply hand cream, comb hair, read, music, pictures, go outside, talk about flowers, birds, the sky. *Trudy, 57, director of nursing, 30 years*

▸ Reminisce, laugh, be pleasant, joke with staff. *Susan, 58, LPN*

What family or visitor behaviors have you observed that are disruptive or upsetting?

▸ Behaviors when the client can't understand why they can't live at home. *Latoya, 27, CNA, 2 years*

▸ Not understanding/accepting the resident's health, complaining in front of the resident about piddly things. *Kalah, 48, social service assistant, four months*

▸ Impatience, argumentative, isolation, lengthy discussions, extreme brief interaction, demanding recognition. *Dave, 40, executive director, 2 years*

▸ Not smiling, roughness, talking down, arguing. *Cindy, 53, nurse, 34 years*

▸ Family being argumentative and becoming frustrated. *Marge, 50, nursing home administrator, 24 years*

▸ Loud or overbearing, taking charge and not allowing participant to do things for themselves. *Ronni, R.N, 49, 28 years*

▸ Confrontations, arguments and being corrected all the time. *Michelle, 48, CNA, 30 years*

▸ I try not to ask questions that he may not know the answer to. *Gloria, 54, CNA, 18 years*

▸ The interrogating. *Susan, 38, R.N., 12 years*

▸ Blaming staff for behaviors of clients. *Edi, social worker, 17 years*

▸ Family trying to correct the person with Alzheimer's. *Mary, 37, hospital social worker, 11 years*

▸ Criticizing the resident and/or their behavior or forgetfulness. *Susan, 58, LPN*

Caregivers say...

Alzheimer's, dementia and memory loss affects everyone differently, and it's impossible to predict someone's behavior. That's why every day is unique and can be a challenge or a blessing.

What has surprised you the most?

- The behavior change
- How well she gets by
- He forgot common sense
- How she's kept her sense of humor
- Weight loss
- Hospitalizations

- The things he remembers
- Her anger
- Inability to follow any directions
- Childlike behavior
- How slowly it has progressed

- When she hit me. *Sylvia, 58, mother, Alzheimer's, died 17 years after diagnosed*

- She continues to have an excellent vocabulary. *Ellen, 69, mother*

- How much joy we could still share in simple things, watching him relish ice cream. *Ann, 49, mother, vascular dementia, died; father, Alzheimer's, died*

- When he said, "Why don't you drive me now? I don't do a very good job." *Edna, 83, husband, Alzheimer's, died 7 years after diagnosed*

- The moments of joy and laughter. *Ann, 63, aunt, Alzheimer's, died 6 years after diagnosed*

- That she can do nothing at all. *David, 69, wife, Alzheimer's*

- His joy when family gathered. He lost his usual quietness. *Marcy, 76, father, Alzheimer's, died 5 years after diagnosed*

- That no matter how confused she would be, she knew to call me day or night. *Judith, 61, mother, Alzheimer's*

"How quickly he forgets, like 10 seconds." Mary Ann, 62, father, Alzheimer's

- That she fought so hard to live. *Anne, 67, mother, dementia, died 4 years after diagnosed*

- What he could remember, poetry, hymns, etc. *Helen, 72, husband, Alzheimer's*

- Her clever answers when she didn't know the right answer, such as, "What did you eat?" "The same thing you had." *Darlene, 58, mother, Alzheimer's*

- How long this is taking. *Nancy, 65, mother, Alzheimer's*

- Our ability to laugh, have fun together, how she responded to me, trusted me. *Gayle, 59, mother, Alzheimer's, died 5 years after diagnosed*

- His inability to "get" his diagnosis. *Marlene, 68, husband, dementia/Alzheimer's*

- His acceptance of this disability, "that's life" attitude. *Marcy, 76, husband, memory loss due to massive stroke*

- The strength that my mom has exhibited. *Andrew, 25, father, frontal lobe dementia, diagnosed at age 51*

- How hard it is for Mom to accept the next new low. *Mary, 38, father, Alzheimer's*

- That it was him who got this disease. *Norma, 81, husband, Alzheimer's*

- She has maintained a positive outlook. Still loves her boys! *Kevin, 45, mother, Alzheimer's*

- How she took a big jump down and then leveled off now for a couple of years. *J, grandmother, Alzheimer's*

- My mom fell one day and cracked some ribs. She was in pain and crying. I felt so bad, I started crying. Even though she didn't know me, she quit crying and hugged me like she would have done as my mom. My mom was still in there somewhere. *MM, 46, mother, Alzheimer's, died 5 years after diagnosed*

> "She threatened violence to 'that intruder,' me."
> Bill, 78, wife, Alzheimer's, died 4 years after diagnosed

Caregivers say...

Was there anything humorous that this person did that helped you get through a tough time?

▸ No, just that he misses me when I'm not there. *Christl, 55, father, stroke and Alzheimer's*

▸ Every day before she "lost" it completely, she would laugh at herself at memory lapses. *Sylvia, 58, mother, Alzheimer's, died 17 years after diagnosed*

▸ She helped me blow up balloons for a birthday party and wanted to pop them all. *Shallen, 25, grandmother, Alzheimer's*

▸ She still jokes about past events. *John, 67, mother-in-law, Alzheimer's*

▸ A lot. He pretended he couldn't hear my mom when she called from another room. Then he'd wink at me. *Ann, 49, mother, vascular dementia, died; father, Alzheimer's, died*

▸ We both laugh at silly things he does, like stacking pans, pouring coffee in the wrong end. *Pat, 66, husband, Alzheimer's*

▸ Dad has always had a wonderful sense of humor and still maintains that. *Mary Ann, 62, father, Alzheimer's*

▸ Sometimes when he was bad, he would start singing. *Edna, 83, husband, Alzheimer's, died 7 years after diagnosed*

▸ Yes, when Mother put on parts of two or three outfits. She had always been so neat and careful of her appearance before. *Norma, 81, mother, Alzheimer's, died 11 years after diagnosed; sister, Alzheimer's, died 6 years after diagnosed*

▸ Sometimes she would just laugh for no apparent reason. *Darlene, 58, mother, Alzheimer's*

▸ He always loved to tell jokes, and every now and then he will tell one. *Nettie, 51, father, Alzheimer's*

▸ When he said there was a horse down the hall at the care center, I thought he was seeing things, but there really was one. *Roseann, 72, husband, dementia, died 10 years after diagnosed*

▸ We played euchre and checkers until about the last month she was home. She didn't like to lose, so I guess she won every game for some reason. *Robert, 79, wife, Alzheimer's, died 6 years after diagnosed*

▸ She would just get the giggles, and they were contagious. *Ann, 63, aunt, Alzheimer's, died 6 years after diagnosed*

▸ He remembered tricks from when we were growing up to use with the grandchildren. *Marcy, 76, father, Alzheimer's, died 5 years after diagnosed*

▸ We could laugh after the events were over but not at the time. *Shirley, 72, husband, dementia*

▸ We would always joke when she couldn't remember something that it was the "F" word, "I *forgot!*" *Judith, 61, mother, Alzheimer's*

▸ Playing dominoes. She "played" her graham cracker snack instead of the domino. *Elaine, 54, mother, Alzheimer's*

▸ He always wanted to wear a tie with any outfit. He had worn one daily before. *Helen, 72, husband, Alzheimer's*

▸ She never had a sense of humor. *Nancy, 65, mother, Alzheimer's*

▸ He would skip a lot, down the street, in the halls at the nursing home, etc. *Vicky, 54, husband, early onset Alzheimer's, died 5 years after diagnosed*

▸ She laughs at the same jokes my children tell repeatedly. *Elizabeth, 47, mother, Alzheimer's*

▸ We laugh at whatever we can. It's how we cope. *June, 66, husband, early onset Alzheimer's*

▸ I smile when I see big clouds. They were important to her over and over. *Gayle, 59, mother, Alzheimer's, died 5 years after diagnosed*

▸ We try to laugh at the little things, not get angry. *Norma, 81, husband, Alzheimer's*

"She makes me laugh every day. That helps me get through it."
Jenny, 56, mother, Alzheimer's

- His smile and laugh were affected by the stroke. It was not a natural expression, but his attitude of acceptance helped us both. *Marcy, 76, husband, memory loss due to massive stroke*

- My dad continues to do humorous things that help us. We just have to look a little harder. *Andrew, 25, father, frontal lobe dementia, diagnosed at age 51*

- Always. We laughed a lot. She was adorable and a very sweet woman. *Sally, 57, mother, Alzheimer's, died 3 years after diagnosed*

- After I was doing the cooking, she offered me $50 to take cooking lessons. *Bill, 78, wife, Alzheimer's, died 4 years after diagnosed*

- Dad is a retired minister, so every day is Sunday to him. Every day he comes out wearing a tie no matter badly it matches the outfit Mom laid out for him. She hides them but he always finds them even though he can't find anything else. *Mary, 38, father, Alzheimer's*

- Many times he is playful, clowning, likes to listen to music. *Catherine, 85, husband, Alzheimer's and Lewy Body*

- My mom joked about my driving near the end, and I saw a glimpse of my mom again. *MM, 46, mother, Alzheimer's, died 5 years after diagnosed*

"She became obsessed with men and clouds. She became more playful, a childlike wonder and trust." Kim, 34, grandmother, died 5 years after diagnosed

Laughter lasts forever

A sense of humor is priceless. It's a lifesaver. It can ease physical and emotional pain. It can diffuse a crisis. It can help us remember the good times and forget the bad. It can change the world, *your* world.

257

The crazy and curious thing about humor is that what makes one person laugh may bore or offend another. For example, one family was caught up in the contagious childlike laughter of a loved one who giggled like a school boy every time he, uh, had gas.

Look for the humor in everyday life. Much can be found by not arguing with a loved one who has dementia or memory loss. If they're adamant that the sky or clouds are red, then make it a game to look for shapes of familiar things and let them tell you about all the amazing things they see. Who cares if you don't. In that moment, you will have created a memory that will amuse you time and again when you need a good laugh.

Find old jokes that kids have been telling for generations. Many caregivers report that their loved ones laughed for hours when grandchildren told them jokes and riddles. Yes, we may groan and know every punchline, but remember that someone with Alzheimer's is hearing it for the very first time.

Look for the humor instead of the frustration when they pull out old clothes that you may not like, but that they love. Remember, it's not about you, but what is comfortable and familiar for them in a world that's not so familiar anymore.

At its most basic roots, laughter can bind and heal us. Engage them in a funny conversation, even if it makes no sense to anybody else but them. And capture the grins, giggles, guffaws, chuckles, snorts and uproarious laughter on video or a tape recorder for you to relive in the future ... when they may no longer laugh or after they're gone. You will treasure that sound, that look, forever.

And that's what life is all about, isn't it?

Caregivers say...

It's not easy watching your loved one disappear from within while they seem like the same person on the outside.

258 **What was the most difficult part emotionally of this process for you and others involved?**

- Leaving her at the nursing home
- Denial and anger
- Confusion
- Stress and fatigue
- Knowing he would never come home again
- What was ahead of us
- Watching her health fade
- Allowing the grief
- Asking for help
- The detachment
- The lack of privacy
- Visiting her at the nursing home
- How he requires so much more time and attention
- How he's mentally not there
- When he couldn't take medications on his own
- Telling him he could no longer drive
- That someone had to move in with him
- Daily demands without the help of family
- The loneliness
- Her inability to make wise decisions
- Losing our "rock"
- How there's not much left of my husband
- The awful guilt
- Watching his dependence on others
- Realizing what we've lost
- Her inability to understand anything
- When we had to sell all her belongings
- The repetition
- Finding things for her to do
- Giving up and realizing I physically could not do it anymore
- Loss of a vital, beloved person

▸ The transition separated my parents. They'd been together almost 60 years. Mom really missed his physical presence. I had to deal with two separate locations to go to assist. *Ann, 49, mother, vascular dementia, died; father, Alzheimer's, died*

▸ I just reached the end of my rope one day and called the nursing home. I had filled out paperwork six months earlier "in case." *Leora, 72, husband, Alzheimer's*

▸ Losing friends and relatives. Going somewhere and sitting alone. *David, 69, wife, Alzheimer's*

▸ Convincing my father that it was time to let me make decisions for him, do his tax returns, banking, as well as daily care. *Marcy, 76, father, Alzheimer's, died 5 years after diagnosed*

▸ Seeing her lose other faculties; she lost the ability to read, to knit, to write. With her hearing loss, we had depended on writing for communicating with her. *Anne, 67, mother, dementia, died 4 years after diagnosed*

▸ My husband did not want her to go to the Alzheimer's unit of a nursing home, so I had to do it without his support. *Elizabeth, 47, mother, Alzheimer's*

▸ Mom realized during the first day in the nursing home that she had to be there. *Jeanne, 64, mother, no formal diagnosis, died*

▸ Getting rid of the home we all lived in, but I realized it was a building and the person who lived there was no longer a part of it. *Nancy, 65, mother, Alzheimer's*

▸ We thought and at least hoped in a way he would be upset. However, he seemed unfazed and disinterested in the (move to the center). *Andrew, 25, father, frontal lobe dementia*

▸ The day we took Mom from her home. We were taking away her independence (home and driving). She was very angry, called us Judas children. She was angry for the first two and a half months in assisted living. *Jody, 47, mother, early onset Alzheimer's*

▸ She had gone from my mom to "my little girl." I felt like I was her mom. She even called me Mom. *MM, 46, mother, Alzheimer's, died 5 years after diagnosed*

" It was worse than death." Shirley, 72, husband, dementia

"I'm not sure if I would change anything"

Sue will never forget an evening shortly before her mother, who had Alzheimer's, was moved into an assisted living facility.

"We sit down to dinner, and I look across the table. She's wearing summer clothes, and it's winter, very cold. I thought, 'That's not what I laid out for her to wear.' I ate a little more, and I looked again. I thought, 'Wait a minute, she's wearing my clothes! I had those at the dry cleaners!'

"So, dinner ends and I think that we're going to change her into warmer clothes. I stand her up, and I see that she's got on my shoes. I've got smaller feet than she does, and I think, 'Oh, my goodness, she's been cramped in those shoes all day.' She got into the wrong bedroom, went into the closet, put on what she could find and shoved her feet into those shoes.

"The thought of her wearing those shoes all day just broke my heart. I called my sister-in-law, and I just bawled and bawled and bawled. I said, 'I can't do this anymore.' That was really another sign that it was time to get other help."

How has she changed since the day she heard her mother's diagnosis?

"I certainly worry about my own future." Three uncles had dementia. Three of her mother's aunts had dementia. When Sue cleaned out her mother's home, she found her grandmother's obituary that told of her death at the state hospital.

"I suspect that it was possibly dementia, because they wouldn't have known, this being the early 1900s. I feel like it's there. I have no idea." She sighs. "I've certainly talked with people about genetic testing, and most of the professionals tell you that you don't want to know. I said I did want to know to plan, but they say you don't. You could be discriminated against on insurance and such things.

"I told my children, 'While I'm in my right mind, it's okay to put me in assisted living. Don't do what I did.' It did affect my youngest son, a freshman in college, still at home, when my mother came to live with us. It was very hard on him. He had to get out and get his own apartment."

"I think my children sacrificed because I was tied down and not able to do things, free to drop everything and run to any event they were having."

Did they understand?

"I think they do. But they all thought I was doing too much and would say, 'Why aren't your brothers and sister helping more?' It was just my job to do this. I'm the one since I'm the healthcare provider. It seemed the logical thing to do," because of events in the lives of her siblings.

She laughs as she admits she had no break from being the mother of teenagers to caregiver.

Having her in assisted living, "my husband and I can now do things together. I think it affected our marriage in many ways. It was not anything horrible, but he was extremely patient, understanding and wonderful. We were tied down. It's not every husband who will let you bring your mother home to live with you, but with my schedule, he'd be there a lot with her, supervise getting her lunch or whatever.

"With work, I was less likely to travel. I would pass up things I should have done. People have been very understanding. I didn't realize until she was in assisted living how much I had been avoiding social events, mostly because I couldn't leave her. You don't realize it. You can get very isolated because people don't know how to visit. They're not comfortable. Those are just little things that happen to caregivers."

What does she wish she had done differently?

"I'm not sure if I would change anything. I think I would do it over again if I was in the same position. My mom raised me. She did a lot for me. As I was raising my children, there was never a crisis where Mom didn't show up to help. When in grad school, I had three little ones at home under the age of 3, and this was before word processing. My daughter, then two, colored all over my thesis, the first 15 pages.

"Of course, what do I do, I go to the phone and call Mom, 'What do I do?' She said, 'Honey, I'll be right there.' She runs here, picks up the thesis, takes the typewriter, runs home, retypes it. She did that for me. Why wouldn't I do this for her? I can pay her back in so many ways. Maybe because of my healthcare background, I think I can do it better myself than anybody else."

She laughs.

She's witnessed a lot of denial in families coping with dementia and memory loss.

"We all have that. We want them to be the people they were, but they're not. It's worse than death in many ways. The body is there, but the person is not. They're not able to celebrate, to reminisce. It's so sad because they can't anticipate anything because they can't remember it's going to happen. They don't know Christmas is coming or a wedding is going to happen. They can't remember, and they can't enjoy the experience because they've forgotten. They're only living in the moment, the time they're in. That's it. It's sad to see that.

"You want to take advantage of the time you have with your parents." She lost her father in an accident and is now losing her mother to Alzheimer's. "Spend quality time with your own kids now while you can. Life is valuable. Every minute counts.

"But there have been the wonderful moments. Once in a great while, she would be lucid as could be. Suddenly, for two minutes, she was my mom. She'd realize. She'd look at me and say, 'You're so good to me.' "

Sue recalls putting her to bed one night while talking about how she was concerned about her pregnant daughter.

"I said, 'I'm sorry I'm late tonight.' She sat up in her bed and said, 'Come here and give me a hug. You need a hug from your mother.' She said, 'She's your daughter, and no wonder you're concerned.' I thought, 'My mother is here for one minute when I need her.' Those are the moments that you just hang on to."

Saying good-bye

"Although in many ways I have already mourned the loss of my father, he is now just a nice old man, but not my dad." Mary, 38, father, Alzheimer's

Letting go: "Dying is not for the faint of heart"

Bonnie speaks from personal experience as she begins an Alzheimer's Association workshop, "The Long Good-bye: Staying Connected and Letting Go." She tells the dozen or so in attendance that as a long-distance caregiver, she had just said good-bye and let go of her late mother who had dementia.

That simple, quiet statement seems to offer an invisible, yet comforting, arm of support these caregivers need to hear as they prepare to write the final chapters of a loved one's life, whether it's weeks, months or years in the making. They are reassured they are not alone in what they are experiencing and feeling, though they would hear some things they really don't want to face.

One man says that his wife is doing better, "sleeping more and I credit the doctor with that."

"What may seem better is part of the disease's progression," Bonnie explains. "It's easier on the caregiver, but they're not getting better." She told of one woman who complained about her mother's incessant questions, and " 'now Mom doesn't talk to me.' We question if the diagnosis is right on those days when the nerve endings connect."

A daughter describes her mother who's now wobbly, doesn't talk much, is incontinent and afraid to initiate a conversation. Bonnie says that the latter is hard for individuals with advanced dementia because they can't remember how to do so. They may be incontinent because of not knowing the time to go. Sometimes caregivers can get them walking by getting them moving so that the memory of walking kicks in.

If they haven't done so already, she advises them to start looking early for assisted living and/or nursing home care and to explore a variety of possibilities. Caregivers must never promise they'll never take a loved one to a nursing facility. They must make decisions that protect the safety of the individual and the caregiver. Too many individuals neglect themselves, and that takes a physical toll. Get on a waiting list and do your homework because the relationship with the facility will be extremely important.

She asks them to remember the following:

▶ *Part of the disease may mean they don't recognize themselves in the mirror. They see an old person, not themselves, because they're actually going back in time.*

▶ *"We know who they are, be the tape recorder for them. Play music, hold hands. If we know it, it connects us. In late stages, it's all about preserving quality of life and dignity."*

▶ *Learn to deal with pain. If they were in pain before, they're likely in pain now.*

▶ *They may be modest about somebody washing them. Based on your own experience with them, learn what to do. Maintain their modesty, and that will get them clean enough. What was their bathing routine earlier in life?*

▶ *Many people say, "I go and there's nothing to do." Yes, there is. Non-verbal is crucial toward the end in retaining a connection. How we walk in a room or our tone of voice is more substantive than what we say.*

▶ *What was their favorite music, not ours. Music stays with us the longest. One man, who had not talked in a very long time, heard his college fight song, suddenly responded and then became silent.*

▶ *Be aware of whether they're a "touchy" person or not.*

▶ *Some individuals mistake a child for a spouse as they go back in time.*

▶ *Take empty spice bottles. Tape familiar sounds, i.e. bowling alley action. Think of what sparks memories to give them comfort.*

▶ *They will have smaller area of perception. That's why eye contact is critical. Talk slowly and clearly. Avoid an overload of visitors. Pay attention if they're fatigued or try to gauge their energy level.*

▶ *Hearing is believed to be the last sense to fade.*

▶ *Things that are instinctive, i.e., rosary, are only comforting if they were before the dementia.*

▶ *The essence of person is still there.*

▶ *It's not unusual to feel angry because their disease is making your life difficult.*

▶ *It's the dementia that may make them uncooperative.*

> ▸ *Coping with these diseases often makes us question our belief system: "This isn't the deal I thought we made."*

> ▸ *Maintain a sense of humor.*

> ▸ *Write things down or you'll forget.*

> ▸ *You're not being selfish if you take care of yourself. Don't be a martyr. It's a gift to others and yourself if you accept help.*

> ▸ *Evaluate what medications they really need. Keep their joints moving to make them comfortable.*

> ▸ *Maintain nutrition until they can't take anymore.*

> ▸ *There is not one right thing for everyone or every situation. "What do they want for themselves because we chose what we want for ourselves."*

> ▸ *This is also a time of grief and letting go. Loved ones experience a loss of many things, a spouse, a parent, a dear friend, companionship, retirement, travel, enjoyment of grandchildren … loss of someone who's no longer who they were and we are.*

Hospice offers various levels of care and non-care. Bonnie explains that hospice does not rush death, nor does it stop it. Medication can alleviate the pain as the body begins its final decline.

"Dying is not for the faint of heart," Bonnie says.

Don't be afraid to ask or talk about your loved one, and remember that funerals or celebrations of life are not about the deceased but for the living, those left behind. If a relationship was troubled, there will likely be more grief and guilt.

Our American culture thinks we should get "back to normal" in the usual three-day bereavement leave from work. But this experience and death as a whole creates a new "normal."

Give yourself permission to enjoy life.

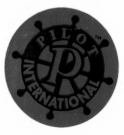

Pilot International is a service organization dedicated to helping people with brain-related disorders.

266

"There is still some connection"

From Anne

When I first brought my mother from England, I thought it was important to bring things that she would remember and be familiar with, i.e., sugar dish, milk pitcher, her linens and quilt. Things that had been her mother's. I was glad that I did this.

Because of her medical needs and the fact that we had no insurance, I was particularly grateful to physicians who took time to understand our situation and act compassionately.

When toward the end I suddenly had some doubts about my ability to handle her pain management, I shared my doubts with a physician who deals with geriatric/dementia care. He listened and provided useful insight and advice.

My sister and mother had had a lifetime of friction and anger, and my sister did not choose to mend any fences. But our mother was unaware of that and did recognize her briefly, and I think she was satisfied that she saw her.

I have found it much harder to deal with the situation of a dear friend, not much older than myself, who was diagnosed with Alzheimer's 12 years ago. She has been in a care facility for eight years and for the last three years has not known me.

When I visit, I believe that there is still some kind of connection/recognition that exists between us, and so I still visit. But I feel guilty that I "don't go often enough" or "can't do anything to help her." The professional part of me knows rationally that I do all I can, but my heart aches for her. The only thankfulness I can muster in this situation is that she still has her joyful, peaceful, loving disposition and is unaware of reality.

"I believe she heard every word I said"

From Norma

I said good-bye to my sister by beginning with the day she was born and talked to her of her beautiful life. How from the first we were blessed with family and friends and how many were waiting to greet her in her heavenly home. It was very hard, but the Lord gave me strength to hold her hands.

She was in a coma, but I believe she heard every word I said. Then I sang several old hymns, and her eyes fluttered a little. This was probably 10-10:30 at night. At 3 a.m, she passed away.

Caregivers say...

Everyone says "good-bye" to a loved one at different stages of a terminal illness. With a diagnosis of Alzheimer's, that process may begin sooner than later.

268

How did you say "good-bye" and when did that process begin for you?

▸ I still don't want to say good-bye. *Christl, 55, father, stroke and Alzheimer's*

▸ Long before the end and not exactly "good-bye" when she did not know me. *Sylvia, 58, mother, Alzheimer's, died 17 years after diagnosed*

▸ The last day, more family members were with her and when I was alone, I kept saying prayers and reading Bible verses to her. *Jolene, 66, mother, dementia, died 5 years after diagnosed*

▸ With my minister, I sat and prayed over and over with him. I had to let go bit by bit with every change along the way. *Ann, 49, mother, vascular dementia, died; father, Alzheimer's, died*

▸ The process of good-bye began the day he was diagnosed and is still going on. He still seems to know me. *Leora, 72, husband, Alzheimer's*

▸ When he didn't know me and forgot how to swallow. *Edna, 83, husband, Alzheimer's, died 7 years after diagnosed*

▸ The last day, he wasn't himself. None of the staff spoke of his dying. I never said good-bye each day. Just "see you later." Good-bye seems so final. *Roseann, 72, husband, dementia, died 10 years after diagnosed*

▸ I guess we said good-bye the night before her death. Three ministers were with us. *Robert, 79, wife, Alzheimer's, died 6 years after diagnosed*

▸ I haven't yet. *Darlene, 58, mother, Alzheimer's*

"It happens with every loss, so every decision I'm alone."
June, 66, husband, early onset Alzheimer's

- During the admission to the Alzheimer's unit of the nursing home. *John, 59, mother, Alzheimer's*

- The social worker told me that he had only a few hours to live. I took his hand, told him we all loved him, and the time had come to say good-bye. He visibly relaxed and closed his eyes. It happened 20 minutes later. *Marcy, 76, father, Alzheimer's, died 5 years after diagnosed*

- We haven't really said good-bye, but in many ways we no longer have our mom as we knew her. *Judith, 61, mother, Alzheimer's*

- As each step occurred, I said good-bye to that part of my mum. At the end, I told her it was okay to go. I got my sister here from Australia. She died three days after my sister arrived. *Anne, 67, mother, dementia, died 4 years after diagnosed*

- It has already begun. I often reach over to touch him and tell him I love him. *Marlene, 68, husband, dementia/Alzheimer's*

- It was a slow process, but she made it easy on us. *Kim, 34, grandmother, died 5 years after diagnosed*

- She had a brain bleed at noon on Saturday and died late Monday evening. We said good-bye staying with her and talking about all the fun times while playing her music. *Gayle, 59, mother, Alzheimer's, died 5 years after diagnosed*

- I began the good-bye one month prior to his death. I spent every minute possible with him. *Vicky, 54, husband, early onset Alzheimer's, died 5 years after diagnosed*

- We had a long conversation two years ago. It's not necessary now. *Brian, 47, mother, Alzheimer's*

- We have not said good-bye yet. The process goes on without speech. *Marcy, 76, husband, memory loss due to massive stroke*

- It was going on for years before I knew it. *Catherine, 85, husband, Alzheimer's and Lewy Body*

- I said good-bye in my head when she no longer knew who I was, but my heart didn't say good-bye until she passed away. *MM, 46, mother, Alzheimer's, died 5 years after diagnosed*

"Three years ago. Little could be said or done." *Nancy, 65, mother, Alzheimer's*

"I thought she was brilliant"

From Jeanne

My parents lost their oldest son to lung cancer at age 57. It seemed that Mom's memory started to deteriorate soon after that at age 79. She repeated things, especially the story about when my brother and his wife came over to the house to tell them of his illness. When he died, it was hard for her to comprehend what was happening, but she would retell that story.

I had already been designated the one to help as power of attorney, etc. To maintain her dignity, I'd make out the checks and have her sign. She then started to hide the bills, so I had to be creative in finding them. My father was also slipping, but he was very pleased to have me help. I know he worried so much about Mom. She had a terrible fear of going to a nursing home. I can still see her pounding her finger on the table, "I will not go to a (expletive) nursing home."

I did the grocery shopping and laundry and cleaned the house. My sister-in-law wanted to help, but Mom would get agitated if anyone else tried to clean. Finally my folks did not even know each other. My husband told Dad that if he had any problems to just push 911. The sheriff's department called one night to say they were at my parents' house. Apparently Mom came into the house, and Dad thought it was an intruder and called 911.

My dad said he was ready to go to a nursing home. My brother and I started investigating homes. On Thanksgiving Day, Mom was having shortness of breath and had to go into the hospital. After three days, and thanks to a wonderful social worker, we were able to get Mom into a facility. At first she was in very good spirits, joking with the nurses. I felt a bit relieved.

The next morning when I visited she said, "Is this where I am going to have to be?" I said yes, and she cried a little. It wasn't very long before she entered the Alzheimer's wing. My dad came to the same facility a few weeks later, though they had separate rooms. He always wanted to see her, but she wasn't very nice.

Several weeks later, the home had a family night, and I took both of them. The minute my mom heard the music, she started dancing. She grabbed Dad, they danced, and she then took turns with other people. It was so emotional for me because my parents rarely ever did anything social together. I remember them telling me that when they were first married, they would go uptown on Saturday night and dance, even taking my older brother along in his buggy.

Within the first six months there, Mom started acting mean, especially toward me. At first it was hard, but I decided to stay positive. She eventually didn't even know who I was. One time I had a blazer on, and she thought I was a minister. I went along with it and asked if she believed. She said she did and was going to heaven.

Eventually she needed advanced care. She loved the nurses and helpers and was very happy. When I visited, she would still get angry. Once she told me she didn't know who I was. I said I was her daughter, and she replied, "No, you're not, I wouldn't have a daughter like you." I would occasionally get frustrated and say nasty things to her – "You are just an old bag" — that would tick her off. The hardest thing was when I was diagnosed with breast cancer, and I wanted to talk to my mom. I told her that I was having surgery, and she told me to quit talking so silly.

My husband was my rock during this time. I just did what I felt I had to do. I would go to the home at least three to four times a week. I thought I could accept all of this because it was something I was able to do and a chance to repay Mom for all the sacrifices she made for me. My daughter was faithful about visiting and brought her son. My son did not visit very often, and I did not say a word because everyone has to handle these things their own way.

I do not think Mom had a definite diagnosis of Alzheimer's. About two years before she went into the home, her family doctor did a dementia test and asked her questions about how many months in the year, the name of the president, etc. He then told her to write a sentence. She wrote, "This is the dumbest thing I have ever done." I thought she was brilliant. Sometimes I thought she was just pulling our leg, but she wasn't.

After four and a half years, she passed away. It was hard to watch her die, but her death was somewhat easier, I think, because I had done my grieving when she mentally left us. I always appreciated the nursing staff, especially the aides who loved her. It always made me feel very secure but also somewhat guilty that I didn't do enough.

Coping with Alzheimer's in a loved one is difficult. I wish that I would have taken the time to do more research, but it seemed that I just was living through it and accepting what was happening. Maybe that was my form of coping or denial. I think now that I am worried that it might happen to me. One thing that everyone can do is to keep active physically and mentally. I have already gone into that mode since my breast cancer.

For caregivers, the best advice is to do what you can for your loved one but do even more for yourself – stress can ruin your health, and this is one of the most stressful things most of us will ever experience.

"My grandmother was a thief!"

From Stephanie

As a young child, I was so fortunate to see my grandma and grandpa every week. Grandma was a very loving, yet also quite proper woman. As a Methodist minister's wife, she entertained a lot. As an amazing artist, she painted beautiful landscapes and on china as well as stitched and crocheted. Her cookies were the best I have ever eaten. Her flower garden was the most beautiful in the neighborhood.

She was no wallflower though! She graduated from college and taught home economics for a number of years. After my gramps retired from the ministry, they partnered as administrators of a social service organization that focuses on children. They took it from a point where the state was going to shut it down, to an organization that is making huge positive differences for the community today, including a school that bears their names. She was, what today's society would call, a "Super Mom/Grandma." She had a grace and ability to know just what to say to make people feel great. Interestingly enough, she was also quite direct – an unusual combination.

After my gramps passed away, Grandma stayed quite active. I attended college in the same town in which she lived. I visited occasionally, but not as much as I should have. There was always more time for me! However, in my final year, I called her frequently to see if I could drop by. She always told me that she would love to visit, but she was way too busy, and I believed her.

A few years later, I realized that she had been tricking me! My uncle, who also lived in town, took her car away after a farmer found Grandma wandering in the country and lost. She was furious. She did not let anyone come by because she was afraid they would see, afraid they would find out.

Over time, she started calling my uncle frequently and often at odd hours of the night. It soon became apparent to those of us in town that something was not right with Grandma. My father, on the other hand, strongly disagreed. He lived in another state, and when he spoke to her on the phone she was very good at conversation. She was tricking him, too!

As her disease progressed, my dad finally agreed that we needed to have her evaluated. She was eventually placed in an Alzheimer's unit, and we discovered how she had been living as we entered her home. We found so many alarming things, used adult diapers at the bottom of her closet, dirty dishes in the cabinets, and much more. The amazing thing was that all of the public areas of her home were impeccable. The gracious host always knew how to make a guest feel welcome!

Visiting the Alzheimer's unit was a surreal experience. Some of the residents seemed so lucid and not sick, while others were completely in their own world. The staff told us to make sure that no valuables came with her, and we should mark all of her clothes and only bring easy-to-wear clothing. That seemed so odd for a woman who was always proper. I really did not understand why they made such a big deal about us taking her wedding rings. She was not happy about that either.

However, the next visit, I gained a better understanding. We found things in her drawers that were not hers. When we spoke to the staff about it, they told us that she had probably taken the items from other residents. My proper grandmother was a thief! My dad was mortified. My brothers laughed. The staff explained that residents often go into other rooms thinking that it is theirs.

She continued to slip, and the proper lady would curse like a drunk degenerate. I felt so badly for her. One moment she would be herself and the next minute she was way off. One day, she got angry. She put her silverware down and looked me in the eye and said, "I know I am going crazy and that you are all just waiting for me to die." It hurt on so many levels, but mostly with the reality of the pain she must feel in her together moments.

As I visited, I watched my family disappear. Not literally, but figuratively. History reversed itself. The great-grandchildren were forgotten first, in reverse order of birth, then the grandchildren and then the children.

I wish I had never seen the pain on my dad's face the day he realized that his mom no longer knew him. It was so raw that I will remember it for the rest of my life. My uncle, the oldest of her children, became my grandpa in her mind. Seeing her treat my uncle like her spouse was also odd. He handled it better than I think I could have. I learned a lot about her childhood because time continued to reverse in her mind, and she started acting like a teenager. We were just strangers she was telling about her day.

They eventually put an ankle alarm on her – the kind they put on people under house arrest. They did not want her to wander and get lost.

Alzheimer's is such a long, hurtful disease. She just continued to forget. Forget to eat, forget to drink and eventually forget to breathe. My uncle apologized for her dying on my birthday. I told him it was a great present from Grandma because now she was no longer in pain and was with Grandpa.

Now our family tells the children about what a wonderful woman she was and all the fabulous things she did for so many people.

What I'll always remember

Professionals say...

Professional caregivers frequently witness the passing of life and how every family responds differently.

How can families prepare for death?   275

▸ By accepting the normal aging process. *Kalah, 48, social service assistant, four months*

▸ Allow grieving process, attend support groups. *Dave, 40, executive director, 2 years*

▸ Enjoy each visit to its fullest. Utilize support systems (pastors, friends, etc.). *Cindy, 53, nurse, 34 years*

▸ Maintain an ongoing open line of communication to establish the support that will be necessary when the time comes. *Marge, 50, nursing home administrator, 24 years*

▸ By being with their loved one and educating themselves. *Sherry, 27, trainer, 2 years*

▸ Palliative care, consult through the facility. *Ronni, R.N, 49, 28 years*

▸ Hospice, talk about it, logistics (pre-paid funeral). *Connie, 57, psychotherapist*

▸ Talk to the person, write down what the person wants done at an early stage, not at the end. *Gloria, 54, CNA, 18 years*

▸ Have plans prepared ahead of time. Talk with support groups and people. Have a will prepared before you need it. *Vicki, 56, R.N., 35 years*

▸ You might know this will happen, but no one is prepared for it. *Debi, 48, trainer, 6 years*

▸ Talk to each other and be open about death. *Mary, 37, hospital social worker, 11 years*

▸ They can never prepare of the death of a loved one. Unfortunately with this disease, I find I wish for peace for my dad. If he could communicate, he would not choose to live this way. *Karen, 46, developmental technician, 20 years*

"I couldn't figure it out"

276

Imagine a hometown mom and pop neighborhood grocery store where the owners live in an upstairs apartment. That described Vicky and Tom, the couple who had found great love and happiness in this marriage, the second for each of them, as they lived and worked together.

Vicky noticed that Tom had lost interest in the store he had started years earlier. He was not paying attention to detail, which increased her work load. They talked. She cried, got mad and threatened to leave the business, not the marriage. With their four children from the previous marriages, they had a family council. Though the stress had taken its toll on her physically, she was out-voted when she suggested they close. "They said I couldn't even begin to ask Tom to give up his life, the store." They changed directions. She focused on cooking and catering, and she thought it would be okay.

However, Vicky couldn't ignore the continuing problems. Was Tom having a midlife crisis or something? The thought that he might be sick didn't occur to her.

"I just couldn't figure it out."

One day, they were in the store. "He asked me four times in three hours about going to Mass. The second time, I asked, 'Didn't you hear what I said?' The third time, 'Tom, can't you see what I'm doing here?' The fourth time, 'Holy shit, what's going on with him?' I didn't say anything to anybody, but I knew something was not right. He really did not remember me telling him. I thought, 'I've got to pay attention.' I listened, watched and kept notes."

While out with friends, one discussed a movie about Alzheimer's. "I'm thinking, 'Oh, my God, she's describing Tom.'" Viewing the movie later, Vicky was stunned. She didn't know the early-onset condition existed and began research during the holidays. She casually suggested he get a physical. He balked but finally relented.

After tests, a neurologist finally announced that the only thing wrong with Tom was that he had a "domineering wife." Angry, they drove for 15 minutes before she pulled off the side of the road. He cried, she cried, and he said he would never go back.

"His lack of interest continued. He never wanted to drive the classic car he had restored. He got clingy."

While visiting out-of-town friends, they were teasing each other, and he suddenly blurted a torrent of language "that would make a sailor blush. He had never sworn at me. I was crushed that he said this in front of our best friends. Their mouths were wide open. This was not him. I went crying off to bed and almost left in the middle of the night. None of us knew what was going on, but all of this didn't make any sense … 'Who was this man?' He apologized profusely but didn't realize why he did it." They kissed, made up, went on with the weekend, and it was forgotten.

What about their children?

Vicky says they noticed nothing unusual and "thought I was the one losing it. 'Dad's okay, leave him alone.' " Tom began covering up his own behavior by asking her to finish stories. He could bluff his way through anything. Of course, the kids were only there for a short time and did not see everything she did.

"I got to thinking, 'Am I imaging this?' But the more research I did, I knew what we were going to find, though you hope it's a stroke, a brain tumor or vitamin deficiency. If it's that other stuff, then it's not Alzheimer's."

A doctor put him on medication because he said it wouldn't hurt. However, one day Tom saw a magazine advertisement for it and how it was used for treating Alzheimer's.

"He looked at me. 'This is what I take.' Yes. 'Is this what's wrong with me?' Oh, my God, what do I do? I just started to cry. I can't lie to him. 'We don't know. That's why the doctor is running all these tests. It could be, but we hope not.' That was awful. I wished drug companies had never been allowed to advertise.

"That's how he found out."

Why didn't they talk about it before then?

"I don't know. Maybe I was protecting him until we knew. I just hoped we'd never have to use the 'A' word." The term had never come up with him until then. For a while, he was sad, and her health had suffered so much that it briefly became the focal point. They closed the business. "For two people who always talked about everything, we didn't discuss this a whole lot. He thought he was protecting me if we didn't talk about him."

Looking back, Vicky would do the same thing because it gave her time to prepare for what they would face. Who did she turn to? "Hardly anybody at that point. Nobody believed me or wanted to see it." Finally a friend believed her, and then a relative definitely noticed something wrong with him.

When they got the official diagnosis of early-onset Alzheimer's, she was not surprised but still devastated.

"We came home and told our kids and called relatives. We just spent the evening crying. The next day, Tom said, 'We've got to move on.' So we did. We kept living as much as we could."

She painfully remembers a spell when Tom cried almost constantly and went through boxes of tissues.

"I was becoming more of a caregiver than a wife. I felt like when my kids were small to find out what was wrong. I just felt helpless. I didn't want to burden anybody. Even though they were our adult children, I was still protecting them. It just broke my heart because I didn't know how to stop the tears."

Tom worked for his daughter for a while and did well. Then he started to wander and get lost. She ordered Safe Return bracelets offered through the Alzheimer's Association.

"One night he asked, 'What if sometime I can't come home?' I said, 'This is always your home.' 'No, no, what if I can't come home?' It was like a two by four hitting me. I wasn't listening to what he was saying. 'You mean, if you don't know how?' 'Yeah.' 'Did you get lost?' 'Oh, no!' He got real defensive. 'I was just wondering. What would happen if I couldn't get home?' "

She put the Safe Return bracelet on him and explained it. He balked until she said she'd wear one, too, and together, they could be "special, like nobody else." She told him how to show somebody. He agreed and nothing else was said for long time.

He became even more clingy. Barely two feet separated them.

"I think he was looking to me for protection, physically and emotionally, to finish his sentences for him. He didn't have to make a decision about what to eat. I did because I wanted to. That's what you do for the person you love."

The man she loved eventually lost his memories of their life together. He knew the grandchildren were special though didn't understand why. Sometimes he knew she was Vicky, but he couldn't put together Vicky and wife.

"He had no idea who he was in pictures. He had no idea who I was in pictures. Sometimes he'd call me by my name, someone he liked. He'd pat me on the shoulder and say, 'You're a nice lady.' Mostly he knew we were familiar people but couldn't begin to tell you the relationship."

He had begun to have some seizures. Tests discovered blood clots in his legs, requiring they spend her birthday in the emergency room.

"We spent that day trying to keep him down in bed, under control. He was wild almost. He was hallucinating, seeing and talking to his parents who had died years ago, reaching out to them, talking to other relatives who had died. He called them by name, including his brother who had died two and a half years before.

"We thought he was going to die that night. We pretty much moved into the nursing home. That week our children had their eyes opened big time as to how bad he really was and how deep our love was. When no one could get him to do anything, I could get him to calm down. Even in that state, deep down, he knew I was the one he wanted.

"I called that our healing week because his daughter and I had had a terrible falling out." Vicky wrote her a letter explaining how she was making funeral arrangements for "whenever" and poured out a lot of feelings. They talked about that letter and how "he needed our respect and love."

He rallied and declined repeatedly for a month. Her voice breaks as she recounts those vivid memories. Then he had three seizures and died two days before his 60th birthday.

"I was angry but not at him." Some medical personnel had told her he had years to go and thought she didn't know what was going on. She was angry at them because they were not educated on early-onset Alzheimer's.

"I spent a lot of time in preparation because I knew in my heart it would be soon. My faith ... I spent a lot of time in prayer with my friends." She stayed many long nights, "but I wouldn't trade that. I needed that time with him. I was able to say my good-byes. I truly think that Tom and God got together and said this family needs a little healing. Everybody got to say their good-byes."

She had been in mourning for five years, especially the last year and a half, going home every day and realizing he'd never live there again.

With the pain still fresh, she found the most insensitive people took her arm and said, "I know exactly what you feel because we went through this with my grandfather."

" 'I'm sorry you had to go through that with your grandfather, but you have no idea how I feel. Going through Alzheimer's with a grandparent, I did that, is nothing like going through it with a spouse.' I just turned away.

"It really bothers me when people say that about anything. Nobody knows how you feel. 'Now you've got your life back.' That hurts. That stabs really bad. No, if I had my life back, Tom would be here rubbing my back for me, or we'd be giggling over some silly little thing, or we'd be watching the sunset. I don't have my life back. People mean well, but they don't realize what they're saying, how it affects the other person."

To pay Tom's medical bills, even after his death, she worked three jobs. "Then some people said, 'I think it's great you're working a part-time to keep yourself busy.' I really want to scream bullshit! If I wanted to keep busy, I'll clean the closet I haven't touched in five years. Or I'll read a good book or watch a movie. I work because I have to, but people don't want to hear that ..."

What they can say is, "Talk to me" or "Why don't we go for a drive and if you want to scream, just let it out." Crying is therapeutic, but if you're crying in the shower alone, "you're still alone. I had to cry alone in the shower a lot so that Tom wouldn't see me, because if I cried, he cried. I couldn't tell him why I was crying."

Her advice to families confronting Alzheimer's, particularly early-onset? Get a diagnosis as soon as possible and enjoy the little things in life. Printed on her bathroom mirror is this bit of wisdom, "It isn't the big pleasures that count the most; it's making a big deal out of the little ones."

"Today they know your name, and it's a big thing. Today, they know what the toilet is for, and that's a big deal. We celebrated when he used the toilet to urinate in, not the closet or a drawer or the hall.

"You'd make up the rules every day because they'd change every day. It depended on where he was at in his mind and what you could handle emotionally that day." Sometimes he'd get so agitated, and she'd just give up. "I learned very quickly where the mops where." She laughs.

"You just have to jump in and learn. They still deserve the best of care. He was still Tom. He still deserved respect, dignity, love. Even though I didn't love what I was doing, I still loved and adored him." She'd clean up after him in the nursing home even though the aides offered.

"My advice, what I tell myself, even though my heart has been broken through the disease, his death and the intense loneliness ... I have to try really hard not to be broken. I can't allow the dragon to claim two of us. I work hard every day not to be broken. It ain't easy," she says, laughing.

"I thought since I had been living alone for a year and a half ... I was thoroughly prepared for his death, but I wasn't prepared for the three months after and the intense loneliness. It's the first time in my life I have not been accountable to or responsible for anyone. ... that's an awful feeling. But life goes on."

What would Tom say to a family facing this challenge?

"Tom would say, 'Hang on tight. You've got to have a sense of humor.' That means love, respect ... hang on tight. That's what he'd tell me a lot of times. He'd take my hand and say, 'We've got to hang on tight.' Laughter does help a lot ... love and laughter."

What would my loved one say

_____
✏ _____
. _____
_____
_____
_____

Caregivers say...

No matter if it's Alzheimer's or another cause, everyone copes with the death of a loved one differently.

282 **If you were with this person in the final stages, how did you cope with it emotionally?**

- Take it one day at a time
- Visited every day
- Wanted to be with her
- The family stayed for several nights until the end
- I'm making sure she has everything she needs
- Very emotional

- Prayer and family support
- Acknowledged that he had a full and good life
- Happy that she was going to her place in Heaven
- When he got worse, I was ready to let him go

- My minister was especially helpful. My sister, niece and daughter came. I read a lot on end-stage and hospice. The nurses at the facility helped. *Ann, 49, mother, vascular dementia, died; father, Alzheimer's, died*

- I dread thinking about it. I had a hard time when my grandmother died. *Cathi, 58, mother, dementia*

- He died suddenly. I fed him lunch. In 16 hours, he was gone. *Roseann, 72, husband, dementia, died 10 years after diagnosed*

- I always knew the diagnosis meant good-bye. *Ann, 63, aunt, Alzheimer's, died 6 years after diagnosed*

- It became a medical issue, so I did okay. The end of her suffering was a relief. *Anne, 67, mother, dementia, died 4 years after diagnosed*

- It was a beautiful, peaceful, loving death. She was free at last. *Kim, 34, grandmother, died 5 years after diagnosed*

- I hope I'm ready. *John, 59, mother, Alzheimer's*

- The doctor and nurse told me what to expect. He'd been asking for 10 years why the Lord had not already taken him home. *Marcy, 76, father, Alzheimer's, died 5 years after diagnosed*

- I just kept telling myself that it was my job, and this is the only opportunity I would have to do this. *Jeanne, 64, mother, no formal diagnosis, died*

- She never made it to "final" stages. God blessed us and called her home. *Gayle, 59, mother, Alzheimer's, died 5 years after diagnosed*

- I spent a lot of time in prayer. Mostly I just tried to forget my feelings and tried to dwell on our past together. *Vicky, 54, husband, early onset Alzheimer's, died 5 years after diagnosed*

- I cried a lot. *Sally, 57, mother, Alzheimer's, died 3 years after diagnosed*

- I hope the Lord gives me strength to be strong for him. *Norma, 81, husband, Alzheimer's*

- He's still living at home, but has been near death two times. I had to encourage him to think positively about surviving the emergency. *Marcy, 76, husband, memory loss due to massive stroke*

- I was fortunate. My mom passed in her sleep from cardiac failure. *Sally, 57, mother, Alzheimer's, died 3 years after diagnosed*

- When I put her in the nursing home and then again and again for two years. *Bill, 78, wife, Alzheimer's, died 4 years after diagnosed*

- I watched her take her last breath. Part of me died with her. *MM, 46, mother, Alzheimer's, died 5 years after diagnosed*

283

How I can cope with death

"For caregivers, it's hard to get out of that routine"

From Nancy

Looking back at the process of Alzheimer's, I think it is a series of steps to the end. Some take them quicker then others. Those who suffer the longest are the families. The care in a good facility is very expensive. Those who can afford it are blessed. Those who can't are left with few choices to deal with the disease.

I could not have taken care of my mother. I could not do it physically, emotionally or any other way. I knew that, and it is okay. It is okay for the caregiver to realize what they can and cannot do. Plus I have a husband of almost 47 years, and it would not have been fair to him. I knew that from the beginning. I have a great, solid marriage.

Death is not easy. But when it comes to Alzheimer's, living with it may be a lot worse. The fact that my mom, who was so alive and active and was reduced to nothing but a shell of a person, would not be the way she wanted to live. She was existing, not living. Anything that would indicate life in any form had to be done for her. It was very hard to watch.

I almost knew the last time I was there that it would be soon. I just did not realize how soon. When the facility called me and said I'd better come, I knew. But I could not go, because my husband was just getting out of ICU after surgery. Within 10 minutes they called me back and said she was gone. I believe she was already gone when they called the first time.

The family shed few tears. We remembered the good times and talked about them at her funeral. I did an eulogy, as did my daughter who had lived with her for a number of years. In the end, we toasted her with a glass of Jack Daniels, which she loved. Since I don't drink, I had diet Coke.

For the caregivers, once the person is gone, it is hard to get out of that routine. I have to think about not calling the facility each day or so. I forget that I don't have to go any more because it becomes such a big part of your life.

I believe a cure will be found. They are so close.

Looking
back

"You can't do it alone. If it takes a village to raise a child, it certainly takes a village to do dementia health care." Anne, 67, mother, dementia, died 4 years after diagnosed

Caregivers say...

Everyday life is a learning experience, and some days offer more than one lesson. When caring for a loved one with dementia or memory loss, those discoveries can be quite powerful.

286

What is the most valuable lesson you have learned from this personal experience?

▶ Still learning every day

▶ Dementia affects the whole family

▶ To be more patient

▶ Plan ahead while the individual is still alert

▶ Have living wills

▶ Pre-arrange funerals

▶ Talk over important decisions as a family

▶ How to repeat things without getting frustrated

▶ Everyone says they will help but they don't

▶ Feel blessed for every good day

▶ Live each day to the fullest

▶ Keep a positive attitude

▶ Pray always

▶ Write down family history before it's too late

▶ Seek help sooner

▶ Life is short

▶ Say what you need to say so it's never too late

▶ Smile

▶ Give people your time

▶ Don't sweat the small stuff

▶ There's still enjoyment to be had

▶ That career and personal goals aren't everything in life. That human connections and caring are the most important aspects of life. *Christl, 55, father, stroke and Alzheimer's*

▶ Enjoy the time you have with them and help as much as you can. Even in the nursing home, I went every day and always checked on her care. *Jolene, 66, mother, dementia, died 5 years after diagnosed*

▶ Don't give up too soon. There are a lot of good days in there, and I didn't want to miss any of them. *Jenny, 56, mother, Alzheimer's*

▸ I learned that you can lie to her. *Ellen, 69, mother*

▸ I have to live my life one day at a time and don't put off activities until tomorrow. I might have it also! *Cathi, 58, mother, dementia*

▸ To make the most of your time together and be prepared as much as possible financially, emotionally and spiritually. *Leora, 72, husband, Alzheimer's*

▸ Friends are so special. I still go to a support group so I can help others who are just going through it. *Edna, 83, husband, Alzheimer's, died 7 years after diagnosed*

▸ We need to "live" every day. Don't leave things unsaid. Help where and whenever we can. Enjoy friends and family. Get your estate and personal things in order. *Norma, 81, mother, Alzheimer's, died 11 years after diagnosed; sister, Alzheimer's, died 6 years after diagnosed*

▸ Enjoy every minute of life and the people around you. Show them love and care and hopefully you'll get it in return. *Nettie, 51, father, Alzheimer's*

▸ This person is not the same person he once was. He will say and do things that he wouldn't have before. Try not to take what he says and does personally. It will be hard to do. *Roseann, 72, husband, dementia, died 10 years after diagnosed*

▸ Be prepared. Get information and plan ahead the inevitable "next stop" in the progression. *John, 59, mother, Alzheimer's*

▸ Life is precious and too short. We should live how we want. *Kim, 34, grandmother, died 5 years after diagnosed*

▸ To face responsibility. *Phil, 69, mother, dementia*

▸ How lucky I am that my father was easy to get along with, sick or well, didn't matter. Also, it helped that I had studied psychology. *Marcy, 76, father, Alzheimer's, died 5 years after diagnosed*

"There can be quality in life even when the life has a dementia illness in it." Ann, 49, mother, vascular dementia; father, Alzheimer's

▶ Hope that a person catches it soon in early stage. Find a better nursing facility for dementia. *Robert, 79, wife, Alzheimer's, died 6 years after diagnosed*

▶ There are always some people who cannot face reality and willingly hurt others. *Ann, 63, aunt, Alzheimer's, died 6 years after diagnosed*

288

▶ It has brought me closer to my mother and brother, and it had made me a kinder and more gentle person. *Elaine, 54, mother, Alzheimer's*

▶ Keep active and helping others. Keep lists so that the brain doesn't forget as easily. *Nancy, 65, mother, Alzheimer's*

▶ Keep them close as long as possible, but don't let yourself get to the point of exhaustion. *Darlene, 58, mother, Alzheimer's*

▶ I am stronger than I would have thought, but not unbreakable. *Marlene, 68, husband, dementia/Alzheimer's*

▶ The cycle of life and nature of love. *Elizabeth, 47, mother, Alzheimer's*

▶ Don't take anything for granted or have any regrets. *Andrew, 25, father, frontal lobe dementia, diagnosed at age 51*

▶ Life ain't fair. *Bill, 78, wife, Alzheimer's, died 4 years after diagnosed*

▶ That caregivers need practical help! What would a person do without family?! *Mary, 38, father, Alzheimer's*

▶ You are never really prepared for how bad it will be. *Sandy, 61, husband, Alzheimer's and vascular dementia*

▶ Appreciate the person for where they are at any given time during the disease. *Kevin, 45, mother, Alzheimer's*

▶ I would hope that anyone diagnosed with this would have some loved one be their caregiver. Each person needs someone with a vested interest in their care. You need to use resources available to you as a caregiver. I also don't want anyone else I know and love to go through this. *MM, 46, mother, Alzheimer's, died 5 years after diagnosed*

"You get good at changing subjects." John, 67, mother-in-law, Alzheimer's

Caregivers say...

Part of our role as human beings is to teach and learn from each other along this journey called life. Those individuals who have witnessed first-hand the devastation of Alzheimer's, dementia or memory loss have acquired many life lessons to share with friends and strangers ... whether they wanted to or not.

What advice would you give to someone facing this kind of diagnosis within their own family?

- Find out all the information you can
- Join a support group
- Make sure you've got the best doctors
- Take one day at a time
- You must be patient
- Contact the Alzheimer's Association
- Talk to others in similar situations
- Talk to each other
- Keep your sense of humor
- Seek and accept help early
- Be honest with family and friends
- Get affairs in order
- Stay united with your family
- Provide the best care you can
- Use adult day care, home health services
- Use community resources
- Delay nursing home placement as long as possible
- Get on a waiting list for a good nursing home
- Do everything you do with love
- Put family differences aside
- Have help around the house
- Don't assume the worst
- Take advantage of the good times
- It's a long journey
- Pass along books
- Go to classes
- Be understanding
- "Let me help you"
- Don't abandon each other
- Be kind to yourself
- Don't take anything for granted

▸ As Ronald Reagan's daughter has stated, remember that the spirit of the person is still there. *Christl, 55, father, stroke and Alzheimer's*

▸ Make videos while person is able to talk and know who she is and who you are. *Sylvia, 58, mother, Alzheimer's, died 17 years after diagnosed*

▸ Try to understand that the person is more confused than you. Just give them lots of love because they deserve it and so do you. *Shallen, 25, grandmother, Alzheimer's*

▸ Don't be afraid to talk about the disease. Tell your friends and family about what changes are coming and how to communicate. Learn about the disease. It requires planning and insights from others. Treat the person with dignity and respect. And laugh; it's better than crying. *Ann, 49, mother, vascular dementia, died; father, Alzheimer's, died*

▸ I would advise them to keep living, go to the movies, dine out with friends and include your loved one every chance you can. It's not over yet. You will never regret it. *Jenny, 56, mother, Alzheimer's*

▸ Give the caregiver paid nights or days off when needed, i.e., a dinner, trip to a spa, a membership to a gym and/or health club. And if possible, pay for health insurance for caregiver. *Nettie, 51, father, Alzheimer's*

▸ When he says something that is not right, let it go unless it's a danger to him. He wrecked our car. I could not allow him to drive again. That was very hard. *Roseann, 72, husband, dementia, died 10 years after diagnosed*

▸ Patience and do not push or frustrate them. They have a one-track mind, so don't distract them if they are doing something. *Maxine, 77, husband, Alzheimer's*

▸ Get everyone involved, get professional help for care planning if necessary. *Anne, 67, mother, dementia, died 4 years after diagnosed*

"Be open and honest with your feelings and what you can do to help or not do." Laurie, 47, father, dementia

▶ You can tell them what to expect from what you experienced, but I think it is different with different people. She was never mean. Try to catch it early. I think any change should be checked. I think if we had a different doctor at the start, we would have have been better, but who knows. *Robert, 79, wife, Alzheimer's, died 6 years after diagnosed*

▶ Keep an open and accepting frame of mind. Educate yourself on the disease and local services. Have a family conference. Include the person diagnosed as much as possible in making plans and decisions. Be prepared for "bumps in the road." *Marcy, 76, father, Alzheimer's, died 5 years after diagnosed*

▶ Don't try to do it alone or keep them home too long before making the dreadful decision to get them in a nursing home. Your own health will fail. *Shirley, 72, husband, dementia*

▶ Seek medical help and counseling early. Try to slow down the activities of the household and eliminate things that add to confusion. *Helen, 72, husband, Alzheimer's*

▶ Sit down as a family with the patient and make a plan that everyone agrees to before it gets more difficult. *Nancy, 65, mother, Alzheimer's*

▶ Take one day at a time. Talk with friends often, laugh when you can and do as much together that's fun for as long as you can. *Marlene, 68, husband, dementia/ Alzheimer's*

▶ There are lots of very bad people out there who prey on older people. The time prior to diagnosis is a great time for unscrupulous people to usurp them. Somehow the word gets out and lots of people try to get involved. Mom got swindled. *Kevin, 45, mother, Alzheimer's*

▶ Educate yourself. Contact professionals for advice. If you have someone to help you, let them, continue to love and show it any way they respond to. *Gayle, 59, mother, Alzheimer's, died 5 years after diagnosed*

"Do what is best for the afflicted person, not what you or anyone else wants." Ann, 63, aunt, Alzheimer's, died 6 years after diagnosed

292

- Plan early, get all the facts early and have scheduled family conferences. Extended family doesn't really understand until they live with that person. *Sandy, 61, husband, Alzheimer's and vascular dementia*

- Take care of yourself as a caregiver and try to "mend fences" within your inner circle of family and friends. *Vicky, 54, husband, early onset Alz-heimer's, died 5 years after diagnosed*

- That there is hope. Lots of people get through similar situations, and as hard as it can seem, you become much stronger as a result. *Andrew, 25, father, frontal lobe dementia, diagnosed at age 51*

- Have your house in order. Network with family, friends, Alzheimer's Association; ask for specific help, then people know exactly what you need. *Mary, 38, father, Alzheimer's*

- Trust in the Lord, ask Him for wisdom and help. Plan activities to save steps and energy. Be flexible. *Catherine, 85, husband, Alzheimer's and Lewy Body*

- Be strong after the first shock is over. Never try to argue with or change the patient's mind about something. They can't see two sides. *Norma, 81, husband, Alzheimer's*

- Be aware that you can't always count on family members to be there for you (the caregiver). If you are a caregiver, take care of yourself first or you won't be able to give care. Know your limits. Don't try to be a super caregiver. Take advantage of resources in the community. Find out what you're in for before your loved one reaches a stage of Alzheimer's. Read up on Alzheimer's, but be aware that the books don't cover it all. Some things must be learned by doing or experience. *MM, 46, mother, Alzheimer's, died 5 years after diagnosed*

"It will be much easier if the family can work together and give the primary caregiver as many breaks as possible." Darlene, 58, mother, Alzheimer's

Caregivers say...

Hindsight is a multi-faceted tool. It can educate us and perhaps provoke some guilt. The distance of time from an event or situation can also open our eyes to things or opportunities we missed or reaffirm that we did the right thing with all the knowledge we had at the time. It can provide powerful insight to share with others. Most of all, it proves that we never know how we'll react to a crisis until we actually go through it.

What do you wish you had done or said done differently?

▸ Been more patient

▸ Been referred to the aging clinic sooner

▸ Gotten a definite diagnosis sooner

▸ Stopped him from driving earlier

▸ Kept him out of the nursing home longer

▸ Made the transition from independent to assisted living sooner

▸ Not gotten angry at her

▸ Not moved her into our home

▸ Worked harder to get more family members involved

▸ Spent more time with her

▸ Recognized the signs sooner

▸ Taken her to adult day care sooner

▸ Nothing

▸ Not had a feeding tube after her first stroke. *Sylvia, 58, mother, Alzheimer's, died 17 years after diagnosed*

▸ I still wish we had gotten a second opinion; however, that is purely wishful thinking. *Shallen, 25, grandmother, Alzheimer's*

▸ I wish I had forced her to a doctor earlier, but we did get her to the doctor by lying. *John, 67, mother-in-law, Alzheimer's*

▸ Insisted on meds earlier, especially those to treat depression. *Ann, 49, mother, vascular dementia, died; father, Alzheimer's, died*

▸ I tend to push him to keep trying. I've had to learn the signals when he's having a bad day and not push him. *Pat, 66, husband, Alzheimer's*

- I wish I'd not given Dad so much information so fast. I learned to pace it. *Cathi, 58, mother, dementia*

- If financial conditions were different, I might have retired earlier. Hard to say. *Robert, 79, wife, Alzheimer's, died 6 years after diagnosed*

- Wished we lived in a one-floor house. He fell down our steps, and I still feel guilty about that. *Marcy, 76, father, Alzheimer's, died 5 years after diagnosed*

- I did everything I possibly could for as long as I could. Retired earlier. *Shirley, 72, husband, dementia*

- Talked with our children more honestly about how things were. *Marlene, 68, husband, dementia/Alzheimer's*

- I wish that we had realized how far along he really was and known that the full-care facility was going to be most comfortable for him. *Andrew, 25, father, frontal lobe dementia, diagnosed at age 51*

- Got her involved with an adult group. She wouldn't join anything, and I didn't insist. *Sally, 57, mother, Alzheimer's, died 3 years after diagnosed*

- Had Dad tell Mom what he told some of us kids, "When I get really bad, don't let Mom take care of me." *Mary, 38, father, Alzheimer's*

- Settled legal questions sooner, talked about it together. We were both in denial, I think, at the beginning. *Catherine, 85, husband, Alzheimer's and Lewy Body*

- I wish I had asked my mom questions about so many things, unfortunately questions that will never get answers now. I probably also would have begun full-time care of her sooner. Also would have gotten my help in order sooner. *MM, 46, mother, Alzheimer's, died 5 years after diagnosed*

"Taken more time to be with Mom while she was knew who I was." *Jeanne, 64, mother, no formal diagnosis*

Caregivers say...

Coping with diseases like Alzheimer's, dementia and memory loss can affect caregivers and family members in ways they may not realize until much later. Your attitude can make it a positive or negative experience.

Looking back, what part of the experience has had the greatest and long-term effect on your family?

- Learning to spend more time with her before her condition worsened
- Learning to be patient
- Never arguing
- Brought us closer together as a family
- Better communication out of necessity
- Financial difficulty
- Guilt of those who couldn't offer much assistance
- Learning to enjoy life
- Taught us how to focus on someone else and not on our busy lives
- Taking care of my own health
- The beginning and end
- Loss of a loving person
- Hoping no one ever suffers from it again

- It has left a great sadness and longing for the person that I once knew. *Mary Ann, 62, father, Alzheimer's*

- I now work full-time on training for nurses specializing in dementia care and in facilities where people with dementia go. *Ann, 49, mother, vascular dementia, died; father, Alzheimer's, died*

- I think knowing we gave her a place to call home and having her become a part of our circle with our friends. *Jenny, 56, mother, Alzheimer's*

"Closer than before. We are all working together and supporting each other." Laurie, 47, father, dementia

▸ We became closer. Each one appreciated the ability we have. *Norma, 81, mother, Alzheimer's, died 11 years after diagnosed; sister, Alzheimer's, died 6 years after diagnosed*

▸ The knowledge she had great care. *Ann, 63, aunt, Alzheimer's, died 6 years after diagnosed*

▸ Including the younger generation in family conferences. It binds them together in mutual support. *Marcy, 76, father, Alzheimer's, died 5 years after diagnosed*

▸ That we were able to lovingly care for my mother, their grandmother, great-grandmother. Everyone learned they had a part to play and a personal gift to offer. *Anne, 67, mother, dementia, died 4 years after diagnosed*

▸ We lost our father after a brief illness. That was hard, but we lose a little part of our mother each day. That is worse. *Elaine, 54, mother, Alzheimer's*

▸ I have not forced my adult children to visit their grandmother. I think that is a choice. Each family member must deal with this on their own terms. There is no right or wrong. Going to visit or not going to visit makes no difference. If people choose to remember her as she was at home, baking, cooking, around the pool, etc., I never had a problem with that. Allow family members to decide that for themselves. I think forcing younger children like great-grandchildren to go to the nursing home and seeing her as she is now is a mistake. If she had a broken leg, that would be one thing, but not being able to talk or respond would be hard to understand. It is for us. *Nancy, 65, mother, Alzheimer's*

▸ Showed importance of family and also, sadly, how even some family cannot be trusted and will try to take advantage of a person with dementia. *Jody, 47, mother, early onset Alzheimer's*

▸ I learned love and compassion for the elderly, a peace in my heart from the entire experience, gives me a warm fuzzy. *Gayle, 59, mother, Alzheimer's, died 5 years after diagnosed*

"It has been hard for the children and grandchildren to watch him go downhill." Helen, 72, husband, Alzheimer's

Just talking...

(Caregiver and client responses and reactions are in italics.)
Alzheimer's Association facilitators Alisha and Bonnie ask if anyone has any announcements during one of the final educational group meetings.

A client says he has a new grandbaby, but "I forgot the name." His wife says, "It was Friday morning." He looks at her and says, "Her name was not Friday Morning ..."

They do not waste a moment on this fall evening because the holidays are almost here, bringing bundles of new concerns, challenges and blessings.

One family has decided to have Thanksgiving at the parents' home and Christmas at an adult child's house because of the increased noise and chaos.

"It's hard for me because it's always been at our house."

"I'm cooking differently, cooking ahead what can be frozen. He does well with all the confusion."

"This is just the way it is," Bonnie says. She encourages them to send out a letter ahead of time, announcing that, "Since you were here last year, you may notice some changes ..." She also recommends they let family know that they're done collecting certain items or not to worry about any gift at all, if they choose.

A client doesn't like that approach and says, "I want presents ..."

As they break into groups, this session is particularly hard for the caregivers as they face several realities, the first being that their loved ones' social and memory skills are continuing to decline. They're not newly diagnosed anymore, the condition that brought them to this group in the beginning. The second is the knowledge that these individuals have bonded out of a desire to learn from and lean upon each other when no one else seems to understand ...

There's a fine line between education and support. With Alzheimer's, it's almost impossible to distinguish between the two.

The formal gatherings are ending but not before they've pledged to keep meeting monthly for dinner or possibly at the adult day care center with their loved ones.

Bonnie nods. She's witnessed the pain of so many families, and more enter the front door every day.

"I look forward to the meetings because I really need to say these things to someone who understands."

"We can talk in here. Half my family doesn't want to admit the problem. They think you're lying and making this up."

Medications are prolonging the clients' cognitive stages more than anticipated, Bonnie says. The public needs to adjust its thinking that Alzheimer's is a disease people die from and understand that it is a disease they live with. Individuals are diagnosed much sooner thanks to better assessment and diagnostic tools.

Despite the weighty topics, this group still remembers how to laugh ...

One couple went shopping, and she asked her husband to unpack the groceries. She stepped outside and when she returned, every box and bag was opened, their contents visible ... just like she told him to. "I know I did," she says as she leads the laughter.

The lesson? Be careful of what you ask for and remember to separate abstract comments to more concrete descriptions.

One told her husband to move a box. He got distracted, and it was later found in the trash.

"We're always hunting for something."

Yes, it's a scavenger hunt every day, Bonnie says. Hearing aids, glasses, everything. Keep the good jewelry out of their reach. Get a cheap imitation if they insist on wearing it.

Alisha drops in to let the caregivers know the clients are ready to go. She hands Bonnie a stack of release forms, explaining that she had asked them to put their John Hancock on them.

One of the clients had signed, "John Hancock." When Alisha pointed it out to her, the woman laughed and asked, "Why did I do that?"

"Because I told you to."

A not-so-final word

I could not stop the tears. I knew that session would be the last in-depth gathering I would share with this educational support group. And much of this discussion had focused on how and where we'd meet again.

I laughed when the tissue box finally reached me after going around the caregivers' circle.

"I didn't want to be a part of this group that much!"

It's like a reunion of old friends ... although half the group often doesn't remember any prior gatherings. That's the beauty and sadness of a support group with clients, who have been diagnosed with dementia or memory loss, and their immediate caregivers, who now safeguard the memories of two lifetimes.

What I witnessed in nearly a year and a half of attending these unique sessions at the Central Illinois Chapter of the Alzheimer's Association would fill many volumes ... the laughter and tears, the celebrations and fears, the embraces and anger, the frustrations and companionship. Too often, there were desperate searches for the right words to express teetering emotions, for those with memory loss and those with memories intact. It's an inexplicable and explosive chemical combination of devotion, trepidation and exhaustion.

What I absorbed as I sat in this ring of human beings was a genuine desire to share and listen, to comprehend the blessings and curses, to grasp a new environment that demands constant adaptation. Too many clichés describe the evils of Alzheimer's and memory loss ...

It's all over but the crying.
The times, they are a changing.
It's not over till it's over.
Climbing the walls.
Driving me crazy.
Stress out.
Hope against hope.
Light at the end of the tunnel.
There's no time like the present.
On a wing and a prayer.
Life is not fair.
Love is blind.

"Just love them. That does help." John, 67, mother-in-law, Alzheimer's

I am forever enriched by the personal stories, the primary reason why I created this book. It took tremendous courage for all the individuals who completed surveys or allowed me into their homes. So many emotions, so many challenging hours, so much compassion and love … it was overwhelming at times to absorb.

300

I will *never, never* forget sitting in Joe and Molly's living room and listening to their almost playful banter until Joe couldn't bluff his way through a seemingly simple question: *What was their daughter's name?*

My eyes did not rest upon Joe, but rather Molly, as I tried to imagine the incalculable and endless sorrow that filled her in that moment … *How could he forget that? How could he lose the name of their baby girl? This is not right! This is not fair!*

In that instant, I hated Alzheimer's more than I've despised anything in my life. And I loathed it even more when I witnessed Joe's quiet tears as he completely comprehended what had happened. My internal anger postponed my tears until I left their house, the raw emotion shuddering so deeply within me that I wanted to shout and hit something.

And I was only an observer … not a spouse or child or sibling of someone with Alzheimer's. Just a friend. Just an ordinary human being.

I've been captivated by the realities and emotions of compiling this book. I hope I have opened new and old eyes to the human side of Alzheimer's and related conditions. We must listen and learn. We must open our hearts and hands to comfort those caregivers who endure these daily challenges and the individuals who cling viciously to every memory until these diseases strangle the very last one.

"I'm stronger than I thought." Martha, 71, husband, cognitive decline

The survey responses were moving, thought-provoking and full of raw emotions. I'll always remember the person who fought the urge to pull in front of a semi-truck one day to end it all. I'll forever treasure the one who couldn't stop laughing when a loved one thought her underwear was supposed to go on her head.

I heard updates from some of the families I interviewed ...

Brad reports that he and his sister, Megan, were "transitioning now with Dad just starting in a full-time care facility. He started to have episodes of violence and was very difficult most days. We made a group decision that the time was right to make a move for the safety and well-being of my Dad as well as all of us. We have no doubt we made the right decision at the right time. We are hoping and praying for the best, but it is still a difficult time emotionally."

301

Continuing to devote herself to support groups and other Alzheimer's Association activities, Peg shared that her husband died six years after entering the nursing home. "His decline was slow. He didn't know me for at least three years before he passed away. About four months before he passed away, he had trouble swallowing and then just forgot how to swallow. The doctor and the staff at the nursing home advised me that they were allowing him to decline, which meant keeping him comfortable, not trying to feed him, allowing him to rest.

"That gave me time to contact family, extended family and close friends. We were lucky because all three of my children and eight grandchildren got a chance to say good-bye. The text of his service concentrated on the fact that he gained his freedom from Alzheimer's on Independence Day ..."

A few weeks before completing this book, I attended the funeral of one of the clients from the support group. Cancer had claimed Ed, who also had stroke-related dementia. A few days earlier, his wife, Shirley, had attended the monthly dinner gathering of the support group members. I asked about Ed, and she said he was home under hospice care, and that her children had told her to get out of the house for awhile to see her friends.

I asked Shirley how she was coping. It had been difficult, but she told me that the dementia had been a blessing in a way. I remembered one of the sessions when Shirley described Ed's reaction to finding out that his cancer had worsened. Then the dementia made him forget. When he heard again later about his cancer, it was like hearing it for the first time, and the family decided not to mention it again in front of him, to not put him through that emotional distress again.

Later that night, Ed passed away with family gathered.

Shirley had told me about a poem one of her grandchildren had written. I asked her to share it with me. After hearing Jessica read it at her grandpa's funeral, I knew I wanted to include it in this book …

Dear Grandpa,

302

*I know it gets tough for you
To just sit from day to day
But it gets even tougher for us
Watching you drift away*

*The cancer that lurks around
Is bringing you to your end
I wish there was a way
To make you easy to mend*

*I miss coming over
And talking about your day
You read the news and ate some
    lunch
I wish those days would stay*

*Now when I come over
I get to watch you sleep
You just don't talk a lot these days
It's so hard not to weep*

*I know you may not know this
I never have been caught
But sometimes when you are sleeping
I sneak in and watch*

*It pains everyone
To watch you slowly die
But you'll be up in Heaven soon
Looking down on our daily lives*

*Grandpa I am scared
That when you finally die
I won't get the chance
To say I love you, goodbye*

Jessica, 13

Until the day a cure for Alzheimer's, cancer and every other cruel disease is found, we can and must fight back with love, compassion and an unstoppable energy and desire to create and protect our memories.

Speak up and tell someone you love them. Alzheimer's can *never* take that away from us … the depths of our powers as human beings to transform each other and our world.

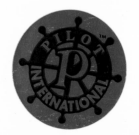

Monica

Special acknowledgements

Thanks to those who helped make this project a reality:

From the Alzheimer's Association, Central Illinois Chapter
*   Nikki M. Vulgaris-Rodriguez, Executive Director*
*   Bonnie Fenton, Education Specialist*
*   Alisha Dault, Patient & Family Services Coordinator*   303
*   Marlene Rush, retired Executive Director*
*   Carla Johnson, retired Public Relations Director*
*   Terri Campion, Memory Walk Coordinator*
*   Megan Reynolds, Education Coordinator*
* · Marsha Ray, Development Director*
*   Jennifer Rose, former Patient & Family Services Coordinator*
*   Chris Clemons, former Program Director*
*   And all the other staff members and many volunteers*
Also
*   Valerie Dickson and Genny Gibbs*
*   Jackie Bowers and Lori Covey, Senior World*
*   Joy Erlichman Miller, Ph.D.*
*   Ketra Mytich*

All the caregivers and individuals who contributed their stories via the educational support group at the Alzheimer's Association, Central Illinois Chapter; personal interviews and the surveys.

Professional colleagues and friends who assisted me along the way: Joy Duling, Stephanie Calahan, Susan Kendrick, Kathi Dunn, Hobie Hobart, Jeanine Campos

And my loving, supportive husband, Roger Wheeler and son, Gordo Wheeler

Each of you transformed my life and made this book possible.

For more information

For recommended reading, resources, websites or organizations, contact your local office of the Alzheimer's Association

24-hour helpline 1-800-272-3900 Online at *www.alz.org*

Also check the BF Press website at **www.alzhelpbook.com**
where your feedback for future editions of this book is welcomed.

About the author

A former weekly newspaper reporter and editor, *Monica Vest Wheeler* is a writer who creates books focused on human relationships, personalities and history, and sharing her passion for these topics with the world.

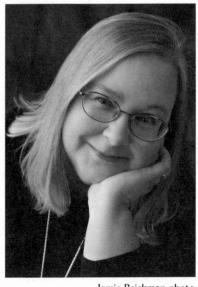

Jamie Reichman photo

A graduate of the University of Evansville, she co-authored, with Joy Erlichman Miller, Ph.D., and Diane Cullinan Oberhelman, the first book in this series, *Cancer: Here's How YOU Can Help ME Cope & Survive*. She has researched and written 10 Peoria, Illinois, area history books since 1994, covering topics from entertainment to medicine.

Monica has several upcoming books on the Holocaust, tolerance, and for this series, coping with brain-related disorders and injuries, children's catastrophic illnesses and injuries, and other life challenges.

She lives in Peoria, with her husband, Roger (and two cats). They have a son, Gordo.

To contact Monica for speaking engagements at workshops and conferences on any of the aforementioned topics, contact her at:

877-COPING-0 (877-267-4640)
monicavestwheeler.com
mwheeler2@aol.com
P.O. Box 3065, Peoria, IL 61612-3065

Check *alzhelpbook.com* for more Alzheimer's related materials by Monica, including audio and e-book downloads.